Eric Le Bourg • Suresh I.S. Rattan
Editors

Mild Stress and Healthy Aging

Applying Hormesis in Aging Research and Interventions

Springer

Eric Le Bourg
Centre de Recherche sur
la Cognition Animale
UMR CNRS 5169,
Université Paul-Sabatier
118 route de Narbonne
F-31062 Toulouse cedex 9
France

Suresh I.S. Rattan
Department of Molecular Biology
University of Aarhus
Gustav Wieds Vej 10-C
DK-8000 Aarhus
Denmark

ISBN 978-90-481-7745-5 e-ISBN 978-1-4020-6869-0

Printed on acid-free paper.

9 8 7 6 5 4 3 2 1

springer.com

Contents

Contributors

Pasquale Abete
Cattedra di Geriatria–Dipartimento di Medicina Clinica,
Scienze Cardiovascolari ed Immunologiche,
University of Naples "Federico II", Italy

Edward J. Calabrese
Department of Public Health, Environmental Health Sciences,
Morrill I, N344, University of Massachusetts, Amherst, MA 01003, USA

Li Li Ji
The Biodynamics Laboratory, Department of Kinesiology,
University of Wisconsin-Madison, Madison, WI 53706, USA

Torsten Kristensen
Genetics and Ecology, Department of Biological Sciences,
University of Aarhus, Ny Munkegade, Building 1540, DK-8000
Aarhus C, Denmark; Department of Genetics and Biotechnology,
University of Aarhus, P.O. Box 50, DK-8830 Tjele, Denmark

Éric Le Bourg
Centre de Recherche sur la Cognition Animale, UMR CNRS 5169,
Université Paul-Sabatier, 118 route de Narbonne, F-31062 Toulouse cedex 9,
France

Volker Loeschcke
Genetics and Ecology, Department of Biological Sciences,
University of Aarhus, Ny Munkegade, Building 1540, DK-8000 Aarhus C,
Denmark

Brian Morris
School of Medical Sciences, Building F13, The University of Sydney,
New South Wales 2006, Australia

Suresh I.S. Rattan
Department of Molecular Biology, University of Aarhus, Gustav Wieds Vej 10-C, DK-8000 Aarhus, Denmark

Franco Rengo
Cattedra di Geriatria–Dipartimento di Medicina Clinica, Scienze Cardiovascolari ed Immunologiche, University of Naples "Federico II"Istituto Scientifico di Telese Terme, Fondazione Salvatore Maugeri, IRCCS, Benevento, Italy

Akmal Safwat
Oncology Department, Aarhus University Hospital, Denmark, Radiotherapy Department, National Cancer Institute, Cairo University, Egypt

Pernille Sarup
Genetics and Ecology, Department of Biological Sciences, University of Aarhus, Ny Munkegade, Building 1540, DK-8000 Aarhus C, Denmark

Jesper Sorensen
Genetics and Ecology, Department of Biological Sciences, University of Aarhus, Ny Munkegade, Building 1540, DK-8000 Aarhus C, Denmark

Alexander Vaiserman
Laboratory of Mathematical Modelling of Aging Processes, Institute of Gerontology, Vyshgorodskaya St. 67, Kiev 04114, Ukraine

Chapter 1
Hormesis and Aging: What's the Deal?

Éric Le Bourg[1] and Suresh I.S. Rattan[2]

Our century allows most people of developed countries, and to higher numbers in developing countries, to reach old age. Thanks to sanitation, vaccination, medical care, and social security systems, we all have a good chance to see our children, grandchildren, and great-grandchildren becoming adults, and they also can see us becoming old, and even very old.

In such conditions, the next main battle is to improve living conditions in Africa and other least developed countries to increase mean longevity, and to improve healthspan of elderly people. This is the job of physicians and of people involved in medical research trying to improve drugs against the consequences of aging on the various parts of the body. Biogerontologists obviously can be of help in this endeavor, but they also have to propose new ways of thinking, in order to discover new strategies to improve life at old age. To use an analogy, it could be said that the best way to discover such new strategies is to think to electricity rather than searching to improve the candle.

The purpose of this book is to try to know whether hormesis could become a means to confine candelabras into the shops of antique dealers, because one has found a better way to provide light.

Hormesis is the phenomenon in which adaptive responses to low doses of otherwise harmful conditions improve the functional ability of cells and organisms. These low doses are called mild stress in the following. Mild stress is now considered by many authors as a gerontological research tool. Data are accumulating showing that a mild stress at a young age can slightly increase longevity and delay aging or protect from a severe stress at old age. However, we have not still reached the time when all scientists accept that studying mild stress can be useful to aging research or even think to mild stress in connection with biogerontology. Therefore, the time is ripe for a book on the matter because it is a time of debates: not too early, not too late. We have a dream: if the functional ability of the organism could be

[1]Centre de Recherche sur la Cognition Animale, UMR CNRS 5169, Université Paul-Sabatier, 31062 Toulouse cedex 9, France. Tel: 33 5 61 55 65 67; Fax: 33 5 61 55 61 54; e-mail: lebourg@cict.fr

[2]Department of Molecular Biology, University of Aarhus, Gustav Wieds Vej 10-C, DK-8000 Aarhus, Denmark. Tel: 45 89425034; Fax: 45 86123178; e-mail: rattan@mb.au.dk

E. Le Bourg and S.I.S. Rattan (eds.), *Mild Stress and Healthy Aging.*

increased at old age, the need for medical care at this age could be reduced, simply because it would be, at least partly, of no use to people enjoying a better health. Therefore, hormesis offers the theoretical possibility not to fight aging by relying on drugs or medical interventions, but to increase healthspan by relying on a pre-treatment with a mild stress. Hopefully, the next years will probably tell us whether our dream was condemned to remain a dream or not.

Hormesis research has a rather long story (chapter by Calabrese) but it has been considered in the frame of research on aging very scarcely up to, say, the turn of the century.

In 1977, Sacher published a review dealing with hormesis and aging where he noted that "the paucity of scientific information concerning the adaptive value of external stimulation has fostered the view that 'stress' is generally deleterious to health and survival". This may explain why the second review paper was only published 23 years later (Minois 2000). Neafsey (1990) also published a review on longevity hormesis, but this article was mainly concerned with the use of longevity to study chemical toxicants, and not with aging.

Reading these Sacher's (1977) and Minois' (2000) reviews side by side shows the main conceptual change which has been done during this time interval. According to Sacher (1977), hormetic effects are "unlikely to occur in the healthy active individual, and are more likely to be significant in the ill or depressed animal" and "hormesis is in one sense an obstacle in the path of gerontological research, and efforts to understand and annul it would be well justified". For Minois (2000), mild stresses "have beneficial effects on longevity and stress resistance" and they "will be really useful if they are shown to confer global beneficial effects on aging". Most of recent studies on hormetic effects do not consider that they can be observed only, or mainly, in "ill or depressed" animals but, rather, in good rearing conditions. For instance, flies live longer in individual vials than in groups of 15 flies of the same sex. Nevertheless, increased longevity after hypergravity exposure, a mild stress, has been observed in these two living conditions, and not only in flies living in groups. By contrast, hypergravity exposure does no increase the longevity of the short-lived mated flies but it increases that of the long-lived virgin ones (chapter by Le Bourg). Therefore, it seems that if hormetic effects can be observed in ill or depressed animals, they are more likely in healthy ones.

It is now more and more accepted that mild stresses can increase longevity, in addition to the well-known effect on stress resistance: for instance, Lamb and McDonald (1973) showed that, up to middle age, irradiated *Drosophila melanogaster* male flies survived for a longer time in dry air than control flies, even if these last flies lived longer in normal rearing conditions. While effects of mild stress on longevity and resistance to several stresses are now documented (see most of the chapters below), less studies have been done on aging, which shows that the Minois' (2000) conclusion that mild stresses "will be really useful if they are shown to confer global beneficial effects on aging" is not outdated. We may feel that showing such effects of mild stress on aging, and not only on longevity, could be now a priority on the research agenda, simply because living longer seems of no value if this extra-life is paid by a longer decrepitude.

Another priority could be to extend the study of hormetic effects to mammals, because most of studies on animals have been done on invertebrate species, mainly *D. melanogaster* and *Caenorhabditis elegans*. In these species, the list of stresses with hormetic effects is impressive (heat, cold, hypergravity, irradiation, hyperbaric oygen: see the chapters below). However, results on rodents are scarce and mainly involve the use of physical activity (chapter by Ji) or of irradiation (chapter by Vaiserman). Studies on cells are not a surrogate for such studies on mammals, because there is a gap between studies at the cellular and organismal levels: increasing the resistance of human fibroblasts to heat by subjecting them to a mild heat shock (chaper by Rattan) does not allow to predict that this mild stress will improve survival of elderly people to summer heatwave. It is thus clear that discovering new stresses with hormetic effects at the organismal level, in mammals, is one of the next challenges of biogerontologists. Whether the increased longevity of dietary restricted rodents is due to hormetic effects of dietary restriction is a matter of debate, the joke being that the two editors of this book support opposite opinions. Minois (2000) and Le Bourg (2003) have both emphasized the main difference between the effects on longevity of dietary restriction and of mild stresses: dietary restriction strongly increases both mean and maximal longevity in rodents while mild stresses have much lower effects. By contrast, Masoro (2005), Rattan (2004), or Sinclair (2005) consider that dietary restriction is a mild stress increasing longevity and inducing elevations of blood glucocorticoids or of signaling pathways responding to biological stress and low nutrition.

We might wonder on the interest to study hormetic effects on longevity if they are of a low magnitude when compared to the effects of dietary restriction (Bertrand et al. 1999) or of mutations, for instance in *C. elegans* (Olsen et al. 2003). The main reason is that crossing the distance between a mutation with beneficial effects on aging and the discovery of a means to mimick its effects in mammals can be difficult, if not impossible. Similarly, while dietary restriction increases longevity in rodents, there is a debate on its effect in human beings (Le Bourg and Rattan 2006) and on the way to mimick the beneficial effects of dietary restriction in humans (Ingram et al. 2006)… if they indeed exist. In such conditions, using an environmental manipulation to (slightly) increase longevity and (hopefully) improve the physiological state at old age seems of interest. If the effects of these environmental manipulations observed in laboratory animals could be reproduced in elderly people, it would provide a new way to improve life at old age, and this, rather quickly. Nevertheless, we do not think that biogerontologists have to give up research on the genetics of aging and on dietary restriction, but simply that the study of hormesis could be another means to understand aging and, eventually, improve life at old age (see Le Bourg 2003 for a discussion).

This book describes the effects of various mild stresses in animal species. The first chapter, written by Edward Calabrese, describes the concept and history of hormesis, and focuses on its use in research on aging.

The second chapter written by Alexander Vaiserman deals with the use of irradiation in *D. melanogaster, C. elegans*, rodents and human beings. The chapter on hypergravity (Éric Le Bourg) describes results obtained on *D. melanogaster* flies. The following chapter (Jesper Sørensen, Pernille Sarup, Torsten Kristensen, and Volker Loeschcke) focuses on the use of extreme temperatures, either hot or cold in *D. melanogaster*. In his chapter, Suresh Rattan describes the effects of mild stresses on cells, mainly human fibroblasts. Focusing on rodents and human beings, Li Li Ji shows that an increased activity level can also be considered as a mild stress with hormetic effects: it is now quite common in the lay public to say that a higher activity level allows to enjoy a better health and to live longer.

The three last chapters are concerned with clinical applications. Brian Morris wonders whether it could be possible to use "hormetic compounds" mimicking the effect of mild stress. Pasquale Abete and Franco Rengo show how better recovering from cardiac accidents by using mild stress, and Akmal Safwat describes the clinical applications of the whole body low radiation hormesis.

As a logical outcome of all the content of this book, a conclusion tries to delineate perspectives of using mild stress in human beings. All the authors of the book have been asked to tell openly whether hormesis will remain restricted to the laboratory or if it could be used in therapy ... one day. The one million dollar question is just this one: "Could mild stresses be used to improve life of elderly people or not?" and all the content of this book makes sense in light of this question. The confrontation of the different points of view could help the reader to reach his/her own conclusion. Merging these opinions into a synthesis thus provides the *current* "state of the art" but not any definitive answer because time is not ripe to give such an answer. It is our hope that this book will encourage and inspire readers to incorporate the paradigm of mild stress and hormesis in their thinking and in experimental strategies.

References

Bertrand HA, Herlihy JT, Ikeno Y, Yu BP (1999) Dietary restriction. In Yu BP (ed.) Methods in aging research. CRC, Boca Raton, pp.271–300

Ingram DK, Zhu M, Mamczarz J, Zou S, Lane MA, Roth GS, De Cabo R (2006) Calorie restriction mimetics: an emerging research field. Aging Cell 5:97–108

Lamb MJ, McDonald RP (1973) Heat tolerance changes with age in normal and irradiated *Drosophila melanogaster*. Exp Geront 8:207–217

Le Bourg E (2003) Delaying aging: Could the study of hormesis be more helpful than that of the genetic pathway used to survive starvation? Biogeront 4:319–324

Le Bourg E, Rattan SIS (2006) Can dietary restriction increase longevity in all species, particularly in human beings? Introduction to a debate among experts. Biogerontology 7: 123–125

Masoro EJ (2005) Overview of caloric restriction and ageing. Mech Ageing Dev 126:913–922

Minois N (2000) Longevity and aging: Beneficial effects of exposure to mild stress. Biogeront 1:15–29

Neafsey PJ (1990) Longevity hormesis. A review. Mech Ageing Dev 51:1–31

Olsen A, Sampayo JN, Lithgow GJ (2003) Aging in *C. elegans*. In Osiewacz HD (ed.) Aging of organisms. Kluwer, pp.163–199

Rattan SIS (2004) Aging intervention, prevention, and therapy through hormesis. J Geront Biol Sci 59A:705–709

Sacher GA (1977) Life table modification and life prolongation. In Finch CE and Hayflick L (eds.) Handbook of the biology of aging. Van Nostrand Reinhold, New York, pp.582–638

Sinclair DA (2005) Toward a unified theory of caloric restriction and longevity regulation. Mech Ageing Dev 126:987–1002

Chapter 2
What Is Hormesis?

Edward J. Calabrese[1]

Introduction

Adaptation is a fundamental biological concept at the core of evolutionary biology and the process of natural selection. It is also a central feature within the lives of individuals challenged by daily stresses. The adaptation concept has been the object of considerable investigation at multiple levels of organization from the molecular to the ecosystem. This chapter explores how the concept of adaptation is expressed within the framework of the dose–response relationship and its biological and biomedical implications. It is the contention of this chapter that the hormetic dose response is a manifestation of the adaptive response, a relationship that becomes evident when robust study designs with appropriate numbers of doses, proper dose spacing and a temporal framework are employed. However, hormesis is much more than the manifestation of the adaptive response in the clothing of a dose–response relationship. Hormesis will be shown to be the most reliable and generalizable quantitative index of biological plasticity, constraining the magnitude of dose–response relationship as seen in the pharmacological concept of the ceiling effect and resulting from the downstream integration of activation signals from multiple pathways. This mechanistic framework not only accounts for the quantitative features of the hormetic dose response, but achieves this in a manner that can integrate effects from the multiple agents, thereby effectively addressing single and multiple chemical exposure paradigms. While this chapter defines hormesis as a dose response phenomenon which is characterized with a low dose stimulation and a high dose inhibition (Fig. 1) it will be shown to be a fundamental biological concept with extremely broad implications.

[1]Department of Public Health, Environmental Health Sciences, Morrill I, N344, University of Massachusetts, Amherst, MA 01003. Tel: 413-545-3164; Fax: 413-545-4692; e-mail: edwardc@schoolph.umass.edu

E. Le Bourg and S.I.S. Rattan (eds.), *Mild Stress and Healthy Aging.*

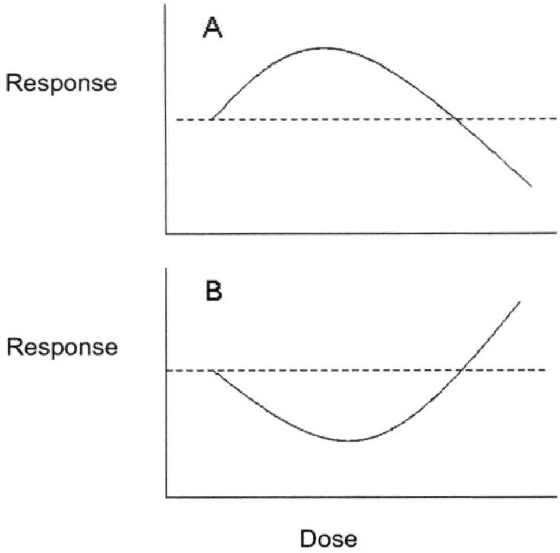

Fig. 1 Hormetic dose-response relationship as seen with an inverted U- and a J-shape

Adaptation and the Dose Response

Toxicology Fails to Incorporate Adaptation into Dose Response

The historical foundations of the dose response emerged from the nascent fields of what we now call pharmacology and toxicology. Starting in the 1880s research began to define the dose–response relationships of disinfectants on bacteria and yeast survival and metabolism. This research soon expanded to include plant growth, physiology and toxicity. By the early decades of the 20th century substantial research initiatives had been directed to assessing the effects of radiation on numerous biological models, including plants, micro-organisms and insects (Calabrese and Baldwin 2000a, b). This same period also witnessed the early development of chemical insecticides such as lead arsenate and statistical assessment methods including the LD50 (Trevan 1927), and, within a decade, the probit analysis model (Bliss 1935; Gaddum 1937) that provided a biostatistical basis for dose response modeling. The first half of the past century also was a period when occupational health concerns became manifest and organizations such as the American Conference of Governmental Industrial Hygienists (ACGIH) were created in the late 1930s to establish exposure standards. This was also the case of drinking water standards for toxic chemicals, with US Public Health Service (PHS) standards being created as early as 1914 to protect the traveling public (Calabrese 1978).

This perspective shows that the history of toxicology was built, in large part, upon concerns to establish doses that would kill infectious organisms such as harmful bacteria and disease transmitting and crop destroying insects as well as exposure standards that would protect industrial workers and the general public from the harmful effects of chemicals and radiation. These diverse toxicological frameworks found convergence in the threshold dose response model which asserted that there was a dose above which harmful responses began to appear and below which none would be expected (Bliss 1935). The threshold dose response model was soon generalized to account for effects that were physiological (Clark 1937), thereby broadly expanding its sphere of influence into the biological, pharmacological, and clinical realms (Calabrese 2005b).

The threshold dose response model was not only a conceptually dominant theme in the biomedical and toxicological sciences but it also affected the thinking and actions of regulatory agencies such as the Food and Drug Administration (FDA), radiation health advisory committees, the US PHS and the to-be-created Environmental Protection Agency (EPA) (i.e., 1970) with respect to risk assessment. Such biostatistical model selection affected hazard assessment testing protocols, animal model selection, study design (number and spacing of doses), data analysis, and risk assessment and management procedures such as the use of safety (uncertainty) factors (Calabrese and Baldwin 2000c–e).

These public health-oriented regulatory agencies had as a principal goal of their hazard assessment procedures the estimation of the highest dose that would not cause an adverse health effect. This became known as a no observed adverse health effect level (NOAEL), a value used as the key starting place in the estimation of a "safe" dose assuming a threshold dose–response relationship. The dominating influence of the threshold model and its incorporation within regulatory frameworks lead to hazard assessment studies with a limited number of toxic doses, often two, but usually no more than three, for many decades. In the case of carcinogens the belief emerged in the radiation community in the middle decades of the 20th century that they may act in a linear manner at low doses (Calabrese and Baldwin 2000b). This lead to model-driven estimates of lifetime exposures, later to be adopted for chemical risk assessment (NAS 1977), that were predicted to cause very low, but socially acceptable risks, such as one additional affected person (e.g., cancer) in a million hypothetical people over a normal lifetime.

While the concept of the dose response was therefore principally used to differentiate harmful from safe exposures, the incorporation of the concept of the dose–response relationship into an assessment of adaptive responses is surprisingly recent. Web of Science key word searching (e.g., adaptation and dose-response and multiple variations of these words) reveals that the linkage of these concepts generally starts appearing in the mid-1980s. This suggests that the concepts of adaptation and the dose response evolved independently over the first 80–90 years of the 20th century. Even the term adaptive response for chemical mutagens was not employed until 1978 (Schendel et al. 1978) and even later still for radiation (Olivieri et al. 1984).

The history of toxicology therefore is such that it became dominated by the use of a few high doses in the hazard assessment process. In fact, it remains so dominated. Nonetheless, this high dose–few doses perspective essentially prevented the evaluation of responses in the lose dose zone, even to the point of denying that a reproducible biological effect could occur below the so-called toxicological threshold. If an apparent effect were inadvertently observed in this zone, it has been customarily ignored and/or dismissed as background variation.

During the early decades of the 20th century numerous examples of biphasic dose responses were published in the chemical and radiation toxicology domains (Calabrese and Baldwin 2000a–e). However, this dose response concept was hard to support unless very strong study designs were employed along with adequate replication. In addition, the biphasic dose response concept became central to leading proponents of homeopathy and, thereby, came to be judged as "quackery" by prominent supporters of traditional medical perspectives such as Clark (1927, 1937) and treated in a dismissive manner. This combination of circumstances effectively prevented the recognition that biphasic dose responses could be real and reproducible; it also served to discourage toxicological investigations in the low dose zone. Consequently, the assessment of adaptive responses in a dose response context was very slow to develop, despite its fundamental role in evolution and human health.

Integrating Adaptation into the Dose Response

Despite the fact that adaptation and dose response were not formally linked until the later part of the 20th century, low dose stimulatory effects were commonly reported over the past 120 years which had the potential to place adaptive responses within a dose response context. These observations, in fact, became the foundation of the concept of hormesis. This reflects a process in which a low dose of a toxic agent induces stress and/or damage; following the damage a repair-related response is initiated which leads to a slight overcompensation and/or overshooting of the control response based on various parameters measured. That is, there was a low to modest (i.e., percentage rather than fold increase) stimulatory response. At higher doses greater damage occurs and the degree of compensation is often insufficient and residual damage remains. The process of exposure and response is therefore a dynamic one in which the organism is challenged and subsequently responds. Since the dose response should also be seen as dynamic as well, it should be characterized as a dose-time-response. This concept has been appreciated for over a century, being best initially articulated in the late 1890s by Townsend (1897). This concept has been repeatedly verified, extended and now is based on a substantial literature (see Calabrese 2001 for a review).

The understanding of an over-compensatory stimulation and how it may affect the concept of hormesis became a central issue, especially in radiation biology. In the first half of the 20th century there was considerable debate concerning the concept of hormesis, the Arndt–Schulz Law, as it was then called. The question was whether radiation and toxic chemicals could directly stimulate biological systems or whether the apparent stimulation occurred in response to damage such as a compensatory/repair response. The intellectual opponents to the Arndt-Schulz

Law uniformly asserted that these agents could not directly stimulate tissue (Josephs 1931; Warren 1945), but rather that the observed modest stimulation was a manifestation of a repair response following damage. The stimulation was "simply" a modest overcompensation to a disruption in homeostasis, not considered important but, in fact, rather trivial. This perspective became dominant in the 20th century due to the status and position of those making this argument (Josephs 1931; Warren 1945).

The beginnings of a re-examination of the direct vs overcompensation stimulation debate occurred in the 1970s, revitalizing the controversy over what is hormesis. In research with marine micro-organisms Stebbing (1976, 1982) convincingly demonstrated that the low dose stimulation occurred as a result of an overcompensation to a disruption in homeostasis (Fig. 2). While these data revealed a compensatory stimulation Stebbing argued that the overcompensation response to damage from low doses of toxic agents was fundamental and generalizable, not something to be trivialized as did the comments of Warren (1945). Stebbing applied the term hormesis to this phenomenon, using the term first put forward by Southam and Ehrlich in 1943.

The key conclusions were that the overcompensation response was adaptive in nature constituting a fundamental process by which organisms respond to stressor agents and damage and that experiments that lack a time component may not yield a fundamental understanding of the dose–response relationship. This is not often achieved as it is common for investigators to use multiple doses and a single time point or a single dose and multiple time points in experimental study designs. Hormesis needs both, making it more challenging to assess.

If hormesis were the product of an overcompensation stimulation, the responses would most likely be modest in magnitude since this would ensure that homeostasis would be re-established with an efficient allocation of resources. Substantial findings have strongly supported this hypothesis since the maximum stimulatory range of hormetic dose responses are typically only 30–60% greater than control values (Calabrese and Blain 2005). These findings represent a general type of adaptive response following the induction of damage with the dose response of that adaptation displaying the hormetic biphasic dose response.

While the Stebbing perspective has been influential, hormetic-like biphasic dose responses also occur with what appears to be a direct stimulation (Calabrese and Baldwin 2002). The direct stimulation version of hormesis seems to be receptor mediated and common, especially in the pharmacological literature, a perspective denied by Warren (1945). The data, therefore, indicate that the hormetic dose response may result from a direct stimulation or an overcompensation stimulation following damage. Of particular significance is that the quantitative features of the dose responses for direct stimulation hormesis are similar to that reported for the overcompensation response examples of hormesis even if their underlying mechanisms were quite different. This is especially the case for the magnitude of the stimulatory response. It is more uncertain about width of the stimulatory zone comparisons since this may be significantly affected by the biological heterogeneity of the system studied.

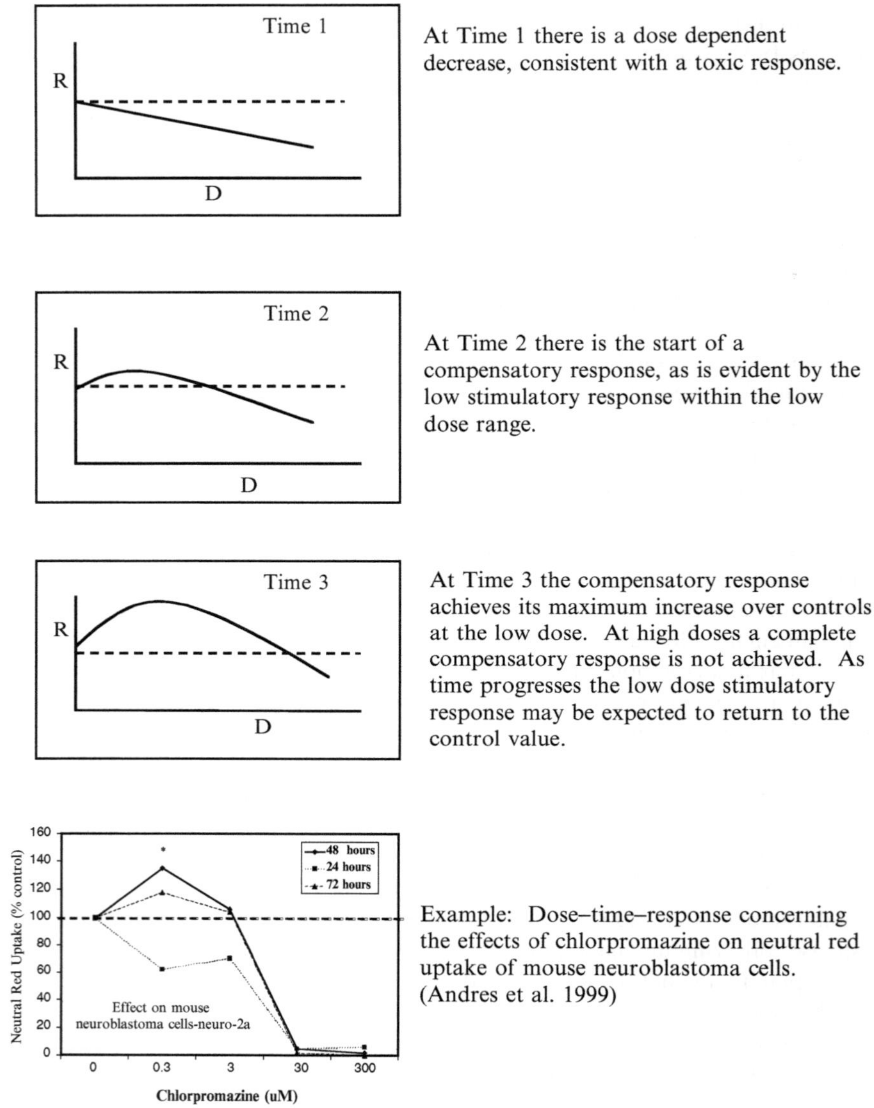

Fig. 2 Overcompensation stimulation (hormesis) within a dose–time–response relationship. Response (R) on the vertical axis, dose (D) on the horizontal axis (Calabrese 2005a)

Hormesis as an Index of Biological Plasticity

The quantitative features of the hormetic dose response are general, being independent of biological model (e.g., plants, micro-organisms, invertebrates, vertebrates, *in vitro, in vivo* systems), endpoint and chemical/physical agent. While the term plasticity is seen as a central and integrative concept in the biological sciences (Schlichting and Smith 2002) it has also been difficult to measure. It is proposed here that hormesis is a quantitative indicator of biological plasticity. It also shows that plasticity is similar across species, biological systems, and endpoints measured (Calabrese and Blain 2005).

This perspective also partially reconciles some debated issues concerning whether a low-dose stimulation is the result of a direct effect or an overcompensation response. Dose responses with quantitative features for what are now called hormetic dose responses commonly occur following either a direct stimulation or via an overcompensation response to an initial disruption in homeostasis. Both types of stimulatory responses are constrained by the limits imposed by the above-noted biological plasticity. This explains why both types of phenomena display similar dose response features, are hard to distinguish without a time component in the dose–response evaluation, and may occur via different mechanistic strategies.

Hormetic Mechanisms

Amongst the most challenging questions concerning hormesis have related to what may be the underlying mechanism. Numerous proximate mechanisms have been published that account for hormetic biphasic dose–response relationships. These mechanisms have been reported to be non-receptor and receptor based. With respect to receptors nearly 30 different receptor families have been shown to mediate hormetic dose–response relationships (Table 1). It is commonly reported that hormetic-like biphasic dose responses occur in situations where an agonist has different affinity for two receptor subtypes that activate stimulatory and inhibitory pathways, thereby accounting for the biphasic nature of the dose response (Szabadi

Table 1 A partial listing of receptor systems displaying biphasic dose–response relationships

Adenosine	Neuropeptides[1]
Adrenoceptor	Nitric oxide
Bradykinin	NMDA
CCK	Opioid
Corticosterone	Platelet-derived growth factor
Dopamine	Prolactin
Endothelin	Prostaglandin
Epidermal growth factor	Somatostatin
Estrogen	Spermine
5-HT	Testosterone
Human chorionic gonadotrophin	Transforming growth factor β
Muscarinic	Tumor necrosis factor α

[1]For example, substance P and vasopressin.

Abbreviations: CCK – cholecystokinin; 5-HT – 5-hydroxytryptamine (serotonin); NMDA – *N*–methyl-D-aspartate.

1977). This indicates that hormesis is not a specific process but a general biological strategy to regulate responsiveness within the bounds of biological plasticity.

Downstream Signal Integration and Dose–Response Relationships

Numerous agents can induce the same biological endpoint (e.g., anxiety, pain) following activation of different receptor-based pathways and display hormetic-like biphasic dose–response relationships. These agents, which have different proximate mechanisms, may also widely differ (>1,000-fold) in potency. Nonetheless, the quantitative features of the dose responses of these agents are essentially the same (i.e., magnitude/width of the stimulatory response). This suggests the presence of downstream integrative/signal convergence mechanisms that affects the expression of the hormetic dose response. Figure 3 displays the dose–response relationships of three agents that biphasically affect pain in the same experimental rat model (Calabrese 2007). Each agent acts via a different receptor, has profoundly differing potency and yet displays a dose–response relationship with similar quantitative features. These findings suggest that chemically induced activating pathways create signals that become integrated via a process here called "molecular

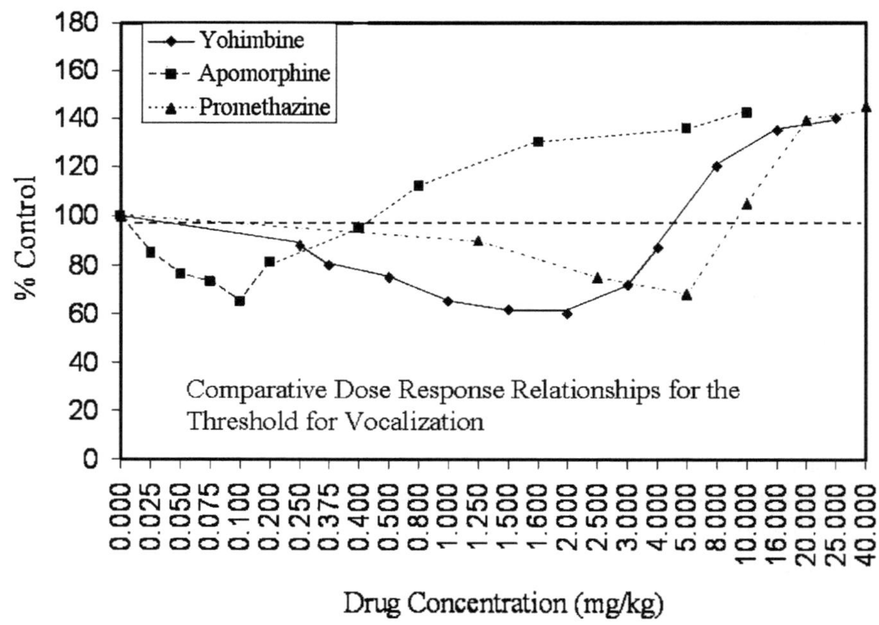

Fig. 3 Comparability of the J-shaped dose response for yohimbine, apomorphine, promethazine for pain (Paalzow and Paalzow 1983a,b, 1985, 1986)

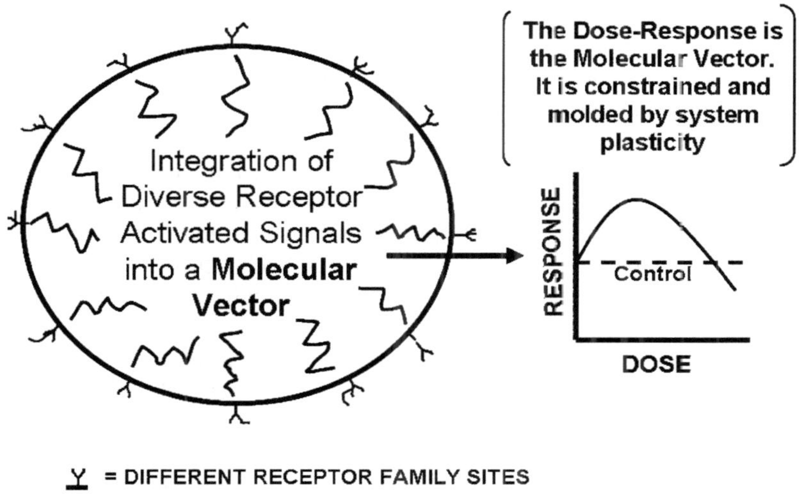

Fig. 4 Carousel model of signal integration and molecular vectoring

vectoring" that produces a dose–response relationship that is constrained and biologically molded by the bounds of system plasticity. A conceptual model of such molecular vectoring can be seen in Fig. 4.

Hormesis and Allometry

When hormetic responses are compared across species for endpoints such as growth, cognition, longevity or other parameters, their quantitative features are similar when normalized for body weight, body surface area, displaying striking allometric relationships. This consistency of response magnitude as a mathematical function of an interspecies common denominator (e.g., body weight, surface area) is a strikingly consistent feature of the hormetic dose–response relationship. These observations indicate that hormetic responses are, just like scores of other parameters (e.g., physical, physiological, metabolic, etc.), in that they can be expressed within an allometric framework. Incorporation of hormesis within an allometric framework is significant since allometric gene clusters are believed to orchestrate the architectural plans of organisms, including plasticity constraints and resource allocation (Gillooly et al. 2005; Ma et al. 2003; Wu et al. 2002), both of which feature significantly with respect to hormetic dose response features and underlying mechanisms. Since allometry is a major unifying theme in the biological and biomedical sciences (Calder 1996), the expression of hormetic responses within such a framework supports its generalizability and centrality.

Hormesis, Adaptive Response and Pre-Conditioning

The adaptive response in environmental mutagenesis, auto-protection in toxicology and pre-conditioning in the biomedical sciences represent a natural selection-based general strategy that employs a "priming" type of procedure to enhance the capacity of the cell/organism to resist subsequent life-threatening challenges from more massive exposures, doing so in a very prescribed and timely fashion. These types of dose responses, as well as the hormesis phenomenon, may represent the same general type of adaptation (Calabrese et al. 2007). Each type of response was discovered independently and overtime a unique terminology was applied to each separately. Since the priming dose that protects against the subsequent more massive exposure generally follows an inverted U-shaped dose response (Davies et al. 1995; Tang et al. 2005; Fan et al. 2005) that is fully consistent with the hormetic dose response, it follows that these concepts are specific manifestations of hormesis. This relationship of the priming dose response has often been overlooked since most investigators have only explored in depth the response and possible mechanism at the optimal protective dose within the range of priming doses. Nonetheless, this concept is clearly hormetic.

Avoidance of Endogenous Agonist and Drug-Induced Side Effects

In the early to mid-1980s there emerged the perspective that drugs that had the properties of partial agonists-partial antagonists typically caused fewer side effects than drugs that acted on the same receptor but were full agonists (Haefely et al. 1990; Jacobsen et al. 1996a, b, 1999). Partial agonists and antagonists often exhibit inverted U-shaped dose–response relationships with quantitative features similar to the hormetic dose response. These observations lead to the concept that partial agonists/antagonists could achieve the same response at target organs, have a broader therapeutic range because of the U-shaped response and have lower risks of undesirable side effects. Thus, the search for partial agonists/antagonists has been one strategy used in the drug discovery and development process.

Since there are many hundreds (perhaps thousands) of endogenous agonists in humans and a general lack of side effects from these agonists in most people, it suggests that selection for endogenous partial agonists/antagonists would confer considerable advantage. Numerous endogenous agonists are indeed partial agonists/antagonists, and they have commonly displayed inverted U-shaped dose–response relationships in a wide range of tissues (Calabrese 2007). While this perspective remains to be more fully developed, it indicates that another type of hormetically based adaptation involves the avoidance of side effects. Such an adaptation would be very significant, affecting a wide range of performances and general well-being, with notable survival implications.

Hormesis and the Ceiling Effect

Since the early 1990s the pharmacological concept of a dose response ceiling effect has emerged with several hundred relevant references cited since that time. The ceiling effect term describes the maximum response and flattening out of the dose response curve similar to that seen with the hormetic dose response. After review of numerous pharmacological papers citing a ceiling effect, there is strong evidence that most have included observations of hormetic dose responses. This observation may be, therefore, incorporated into the broader concept of the hormetic dose response.

The concept of ceiling effect is important since it demonstrates the maximum potential of a biological process. It fixes the boundaries for what can be achieved with respect to biological performance following drug treatment. In the case of the hormetic dose response, the ceiling effect is less than twofold greater than the control response and usually only about 30–60% greater than the control value. As suggested above, the ceiling effect concept is a marker of the hormetically based biological plasticity index. The biological implications of the ceiling effect are considerable since it indicates that performance is enhanced only to a modest degree. The implications of a 30–60% increase could markedly vary depending on the specific situation (e.g., agricultural productivity, memory, hair growth, anxiety reduction).

Conclusions

Hormesis is a central concept in the biological, biomedical, and toxicological sciences that has been generally denied or ignored by regulatory communities (e.g., EPA, FDA) worldwide. The hormetic biphasic dose response is a relatively recent concept in the biomedical community, having received a strong conceptual foundation 30 years ago by Szabadi (1977). Yet, hormesis remains vastly underappreciated within biomedical disciplines, being described by a plethora of subdiscipline specific terms with little recognition of its possible generalizability and centrality as a biological concept. However, there is a growing body of evidence that the hormetic dose response may be the most common dose response model, out-competing the other leading dose response model candidates in fair head to head competition in which large numbers of representative biological models, endpoints and chemical agents have been assessed (Calabrese and Baldwin 2001b, 2003; Calabrese et al. 2006).

The quantitative features of the hormetic dose response occur as an expression of an adaptive response following a disruption in homeostasis, as a response to adapting/preconditioning/priming doses, or as a direct stimulation in numerous pharmacological systems. These quantitative characteristics are consistent across biological models, endpoints and stressor agents suggesting the occurrence of a reliable index of biological plasticity across biological models, at all levels of biological organization, from cell to whole organism. That hormesis is a quantitative index of biological plasticity indicates that this concept is even far more significant than "simply" being the most likely fundamental dose response model.

Plasticity is a very widespread and fundamental concept, often reported with respect to neural processes but also broadly integrated into essentially all aspects of the biological sciences, even on the ecological level. To date there has been no attempt to develop a general and quantitative index of plasticity. That the hormetic dose response defines the quantitative features of the plasticity of biological systems from bacteria to humans and is rooted in their allometric properties is a significant unifying framework with much supportive data.

While the overcompensation concept of hormesis is a manifestation of an adaptive response, the proposal that endogenous agonists have been selected, as least in part, to reduce risks of undesirable side effects and is achieved via the facility of a hormesis dose-response framework is also a significant conceptual development. In these instances the inverted U-shaped dose response displays the same quantitative features as the hormetic overcompensation response because it functions within the constraints imposed by plasticity limits.

Another novel concept presented is that hormetic mechanisms provide a vehicle for downstream integration of signals from multiple receptor pathways. Numerous agonists that act via different receptor-mediated pathways can cause the same biological endpoint and display the same quantitative features of the dose–response relationship even though profoundly differing in potency. This is also seen when multiple agents are administered.

The hormetic dose response, which displays a ceiling effect within the context of the constraints imposed by its biological plasticity, will not exceed such limits. Some groups have tried to create experimental frameworks to create a new "set point", as in the case of addictive behaviors, but this is also done within the limits of plasticity and therefore the hormetic dose-response model (Ahmed and Koob 2005).

That the scientific community can be independently and actively pursuing key biological concepts such as the adaptive response, preconditioning and autoprotection and not appreciate their conceptual and operational similarities and integrative features has been problematic. Each of these areas has their own terminology, research following and educational/society interface. Yet there has been a general lack of appreciation that each area is related to the same basic biological concept and is a manifestation of the hormetic dose response. This is likely an example of negative features of biological hyper-specialization, that is, where a general principle can be missed because the biological sciences have become too specialized, inadequately communicating with and appreciating developments in other areas.

In retrospect, when my investigations on hormesis were re-initiated more than 20 years ago, it concerned whether hormetic effects could possibly occur, even if somewhat paradoxical and rare. However, during this time, it has been learned that not only is the hormetic phenomenon experimentally reproducible but the most fundamental dose response and more common than other models (e.g., threshold, linear models). However, as noted in this chapter, this prolonged and detailed study of possible hormetic dose responses has yielded other unsuspected findings of a fundamental nature concerning its capacity to estimate biological plasticity in most, if not all, biological systems, to predict the capacity of drugs to improve performance singly and in combination, how endogenous agonists may have been selected to avoid side effects, and how biological systems are protected against injury and disease. Thus, hormesis is much more than a biphasic dose-response curiosity. It is, in fact, a basic biological concept of profound evolutionary and biomedical significance that only recently has started to be recognized. It is expected that the hormesis concept will become a widespread and dominant theme in the biological sciences in the decades to follow.

Acknowledgements Effort sponsored by the Air Force Office of Scientific Research, Air Force Material Command, USAF, under grant number FA9550-04-1-0104. The US Government is authorized to reproduce and distribute for governmental purposes notwithstanding any copyright notation thereon. The views and conclusions contained herein are those of the authors and should not be interpreted as necessarily representing the official policies or endorsement, either expressed or implied, of the Air Force Office of Scientific Research or the US Government.

References

Andres MI, Repetto G, Sanz P, and Repetto M (1999) Biochemical effects of chlorpromazine on mouse neuroblastoma cells. *Vet Hum Toxicol* 41:273–278

Ahmed SH, Koob GF (2005) Transition to drug addiction: a negative reinforcement model based on an allostatic decrease in reward function. *Psychopharmacology*, 180:473–490

Bliss CI (1935) The calculation of the dosage – mortality curve from small numbers. *Ann Appl Biol*, 22:134–167

Calabrese EJ (2007) Pain and U-shaped dose responses: occurrence, mechanisms and clinical implications. *Crit Rev Toxicol* (In Press)

Calabrese EJ (2007b) An assessment of anxiolytic drug screening tests: hormetic dose responses predominate. *Crit Rev Toxicol* (In Press)

Calabrese EJ (2005a) Paradigm lost, paradigm found: the re-emergence of hormesis as a fundamental dose response model in the toxicological sciences. *Env Poll*, 138:379–411

Calabrese EJ (2005b) Historical blunders: how toxicology got the dose-response relationship half right. *Cell Mol Biol*, 51:643–654

Calabrese EJ (2001) Overcompensation stimulation: a mechanism for hormetic effects. *Crit Rev Toxicol*, 31:425–470

Calabrese EJ (Editor) (1978) *Methodological Approaches to Deriving Environmental and Occupational Health Standards*. John Wiley, New York

Calabrese EJ, Baldwin LA (2003) The hormetic dose response model is more common than the threshold model in toxicology. *Toxicol Sci*, 71:246–250

Calabrese EJ, Baldwin, LA (2002) Defining hormesis. *Hum. Exp. Toxicol.*, 21:91–97

Calabrese EJ, Baldwin LA (Editors) (2001a) Special issue: scientific foundations of hormesis. *Crit Rev Toxicol*, 31:351–695

Calabrese EJ, Baldwin LA (2001b) The frequency of U-shaped dose responses in the toxicological literature. *Toxicol Sci*, 62:330–338

Calabrese EJ, Baldwin LA (2000a) Chemical hormesis: its historical foundations as a biological hypothesis. *Hum Exp Toxicol*, 19:2–31

Calabrese EJ, Baldwin LA (2000b) The marginalization of hormesis. *Hum Exp Toxicol*, 19(1):32–40

Calabrese EJ, Baldwin LA (2000c) Radiation hormesis: its historical foundations as a biological hypothesis. *Human Exp Toxicol*, 19:41–75

Calabrese EJ, Baldwin LA (2000d) Radiation hormesis: Part 2 – the demise of a legitimate hypothesis. *Human Exp Toxicol*, 19:76–84

Calabrese EJ, Baldwin LA (2000e) Tales of two similar hypotheses: the rise and fall of chemical and radiation hormesis. *Human Exp Toxicol*, 19:86–97

Calabrese EJ, Blain R (2005) The occurrence of hormetic dose responses in the toxicological literature, the hormesis database: an overview. *Toxicol Appl Pharmacol*, 202:289–301

Calabrese EJ, Staudenmayer JW, Stanek EJ, Hoffmann GR (2006) Hormesis outperforms threshold model in NCI anti-tumor drug screening data. *Tox Sci*, 94:368–378

Calabrese EJ, et al. (more than 50 authors) (2007) Biological stress response terminology: integrating the concepts of adaptive response and preconditioning stress within a hormetic dose-response framework. *Toxicol Appl Pharmacol*, 222:122–128

Calder WA (Editor) (1996) *Size, Function, and Life History*. Dover, Mineola, New York

Clark AJ (1937) *Handbook of Experimental Pharmacology*. Von Juluis Springer, Berlin

Clark AJ (1927) The historical aspects of quackery, Part 2. *Brit Med J*, 1927:960–960

Davies JMS, Lowry CV, Davies KJA (1995) Transcient adaptation to oxidative stressing yeast. *Arch Biochem Biophysics*, 317:1–6

Fan GH, Qi C, Chen SD (2005) Heat shock proteins reduce toxicity of 1-methyl-4-phenylpyridinium ion in SK-N-SH cells. *J Neurosci Res*, 82:551–562

Gaddum JH (1937) The quantitative effects of antagonistic drugs. *J Physiol*, 89:7P–9P

Gillooly JF, Allen AP, West GB, Brown JH (2005) The rate of DNA evolution: effects of body size and temperature on the molecular clock. *Proc Nat Acad Sci USA*, 102:140–145

Haefely W, Martin JR, and Schoch P (1990) Novel anxiolytics that act as partial agonists at benzodiazepine receptors. *Trends Pharmacol Sci*, 11:452–456

Jacobsen EJ, Stelzer LS, TenBrink RE, Belonga KL, Carter DB, Im HK, Im WB, Sethy VH, Tang AH, VonVoigtlander PF, Petke JD, Zhong WZ, Mickelson JW (1999) Piperazine imidazo[1,5-a]quinoxaline ureas as high-affinity $GABA_A$ ligands of dual functionality. *J Med Chem*, 42:1123–1144

Jacobsen EJ, TenBrink RE, Stelzer LS, Belonga KL, Carter DB, Im HK, Im WB, Sethy VH, Tang AH, VonVoigtlander PF, Petke JD (1996a) High-affinity partial agonist imidazo[1,5-a] quinoxaline amides, carbamates, and ureas at the γ-aminobutyric acid A/benzodiazepine receptor complex. *J Med Chem*, 39:158–175

Jacobsen EJ, Stelzer LS, Belonga KL, Carter DB, Im WB, Sethy VH, Tang AH, VonVoigtlander PF, Petke JD (1996b) 3-Phenyl-substituted imidazo[1,5-a]quinoxalin-4-ones and imidazo[1,5-a] quinoxaline ureas that have high affinity at the $GABA_A$/benzodiazepine receptor complex. *J Med Chem*, 39:3820–3836

Josephs I, Guido L (Editors) (1931) Holzknecht. *Radiology*, 17:1316–1318

Ma CX, Casella G, Littell RC, Khuri AI, Wu RL (2003) Exponential mapping of quantitative trait loci governing allometric relationships in organisms. *Math Biol*, 47:313–324

National Academy of Sciences (NAS) (1977) *Drinking Water and Health*. Washington, DC, p. 939

Olivieri G, Bodycote J, Wolff S (1984) Adaptive response of human lymphocytes to low concentrations of radioactive thymidine. *Science*, 223:594–597

Paalzow LK, Paalzow GHM (1986) Concentration-response relations for apomorphine effects on heart rate in conscious rats. *Eur J Pharmacol*, 88:28–34

Paalzow GHM, Paalzow LK (1985) Promethazine both facilitates and inhibits nociception in rats: effect of the testing procedure. *Psychopharmacology*, 85:31–36

Paalzow GHM, Paalzow LK. (1983a) Opposing effects of apomorphine on pain in rats. Evaluation of the dose-response curve. *Eur J Pharmacol*, 88:27–35

Paalzow GHM, Paalzow LK (1983b) Yohimbine both increases and decreases nociceptive thresholds in rats: evaluation of the dose-response relationship. *Naunyn-Schmied Arch Pharmacol*, 322:193–197

Schendel PF, Defais M, Jeggo P, Samson L, Cairns J (1978) Pathways of mutagenesis and repair in *Escherichia coli* exposed to low levels of simple alkylating agents. *J Bacteriol*, 135:466–475

Schlichting CD, Smith H (2002) Phenotypic plasticity: linking molecular mechanisms with evolutionary outcomes. *Evol Ecol*, 16:189–211

Southam CM, Ehrlich J (1943) Effects of extracts of western red-cedar heartwood on certain wood-decaying fungi in culture. *Phytopathology*, 33:517–524

Stebbing ARD (1982) Hormesis – the stimulation of growth by low levels of inhibitors. *Sci Total Env*, 22:213–234

Stebbing ARD (1976) Effects of low metal levels on a clonal hydroid. *J Marine Biol Assoc UK*, 56:977–994

Szabadi E (1977) Model of 2 functionally antagonistic receptor populations activated by same agonist. *J Theor Biol*, 69:101–112

Tang XQ, Feng JQ, Chen J, Chen PX, Zhi JL, Cui Y, Guo RX, Yum HM (2005) Protection of oxidative preconditioning against apoptosis induced by H_2O_2 in PC 12 cells: mechanisms via MMP, ROS, and Bcl-2. *Brain Res*, 1057:57–64

Townsend CO (1897) The correlation of growth under the influence of injuries. *Ann Bot*, 11:509–532

Trevan JW (1927) The error of determination of toxicity. *Proc Royal Soc London B*, 101:483–514

Warren S (1945) The histopathology of radiation lesions. *Physiol Rev*, 25:225–238

Wu RL, Ma CX, Littell RC, Casella G (2002) A statistical model for the genetic origin of allometric scaling laws in biology. *Theor Biol*, 219:121–135

Chapter 3
Irradiation and Hormesis

Alexander M. Vaiserman

Radiation Hormesis: A Historical Introduction

Since the discovery of radioactivity more than a century ago, there are mountains of data about the effects of radiation on health. There is consensus that large doses cause harm. However, intense controversy exists regarding the health effects of low-level radiation.

At the end of the 19th century and early in 20th century, it was generally believed that ionizing radiation has numerous beneficial effects. The low doses of radiation, mostly radium and X-rays, were considered to be medical marvels. It was claimed, for example, that blindness might be cured by X-rays. People went to spas to drink radioactive water or stayed for hours in caves to be irradiated by ionizing radiation. The "mild radium therapy" was widely used. This therapy involved the oral or parenteral administration of microgram quantities of radium and its daughter isotopes, often as cures for rheumatic diseases, hypertension, and metabolic disorders. Between 1925 and 1930 over 400,000 bottles of distilled water containing radium-226 and radium-228 were sold. It was advertised that some mixtures could treat over 150 diseases, especially lassitude and sexually impotence. The death of the Pittsburgh millionaire Eben M. Byers by radium poisoning in 1932 brought to an end to the era of "mild radium therapy" and alerted the public, and much of the medical profession, of the harmful effects of this therapy (for reviews see, e.g., Macklis 1990; Wolff 1992).

Soon after the atomic bombing of Hiroshima and Nagasaki in 1945, the *linear no-threshold (LNT) radiation risk model* was derived. This model assumes that any exposure to ionizing radiation constitutes a risk for health and that risks increase proportionally with exposure. Primary, this model was offered as a prudent operational guideline. However, it acquired later the aura of fact even though no one has ever generated any evidence for it. In extrapolating from high- to low-dose patterns of exposure, it neglects the fact that organisms have always been exposed to low

---

Laboratory of Mathematical Modelling of Aging Processes, Institute of Gerontology, Vyshgorodskaya St. 67, Kiev 04114, Ukraine. Tel: +38-044-4310579; Fax: +38-044-4329956; e-mail: vaiserman@geront.kiev.ua

doses of radiation and have found ways to deal with these doses. The *radiation hormesis model*, on the contrary, holds that these mechanisms are always at work and that they are effective against low doses of radiation as well as other stresses. Furthermore, these mechanisms are stimulated by ongoing low-level radiation exposure and thus lead to overall improved health. Only when they are overwhelmed by high doses of radiation do they break down, with resulting demonstrable harm to cells and organisms.

The beneficial and protective effects of low doses of ionizing radiation have been known since the end of 19th century. Soon after the discovery of Roentgen radiation, such effects were found by Atkinson in blue-green algae (Atkinson 1898). He noticed an increased growth rate of algae exposed to X-rays. This effect was confirmed later (Conter et al. 1983). In 1943, at the beginning of the Manhattan Project, it was found that the animals exposed to inhalation of uranium dust at levels that were expected to be fatal, really have appeared to be healthier and long-lived, and had more offspring than the non-contaminated control animals (cited in Brucer 1990). The first United Nations Scientific Committee on the Effects of Atomic Radiation (UNSCEAR) report published in 1958 presented the results of the experiments showing longer survival times of mice and guinea pigs exposed to small doses of gamma radiation and fast neutrons. These results were interpreted by UNSCEAR as indicating the existence of a threshold, but the hormetic effect was not noticed (UNSCEAR 1958). The early studies that investigated life span extension by low level irradiations were based on the theory of radiation hormesis stating that the consequences of exposure to hormetic factors would depend more on the condition of the organism rather than on the agent itself. Hormesis was supposed to enable individuals to reach their maximum longevity. The first studies emphasized that hormesis should be greater in populations raised in sub-optimal conditions, or within populations, in less healthy individuals. They did not view hormesis as a general phenomenon, but as dependent on the conditions of the experimental organisms tested. However, when chronic irradiation experiments were done with high standards of animal maintenance, hormetic effects diminish in magnitude but do not disappear entirely (for review see, e.g., Sacher 1977).

Since the 1960s, hormetic effects of the low-level radiation, which are in direct contradiction to the linear no-threshold hypothesis, have been traditionally ignored in radiation protection practice, even though the number of published papers on this subject surpasses 1,000. During the four previous decades, the benefit from low doses of radiation was found at biochemical, cellular, and organismic levels, in cell cultures, microorganisms, plants, invertebrates, and animals. Many physiologic functions show radiation hormesis: growth, cell division, enzyme induction, metabolism, neuromuscular development, hearing and visual acuity, learning and memory. In mammals, radiation hormesis enhances defence reactions against neoplastic and infectious diseases, improves fertility, and increases longevity (Luckey 1991, 1999).

During the long period of time from the 1950s up to the beginning of the 1980s, four major hypotheses were discussed that explain the health benefits and life span extension in response to a recognized injurious treatment. According to these hypotheses, radiation:

(1) Reduces the number of harmful bacteria in the organism (Sacher 1956; Sacher 1963)
(2) Inactivates gonadal function resulting in conservation of resources (Sullivan and Grosch 1963; Lamb 1964; Hunter and Krithayakiern 1971)
(3) Reduces the rate of oxygen consumption and, hence, metabolic activity (Allen and Sohal 1982)
(4) Induces an over-compensatory repair mechanism (Cork 1957; Carlson and Jackson 1959)

Currently, only the last hypothesis is in a focus of attention. Now, at the top of the list of these mechanisms are changes in gene expression, stimulation of DNA repair, production of stress proteins, detoxication of free radicals, activation of membrane receptors and release of growth factors, stimulation of the immunological system, and compensatory cell proliferation (for reviews see Luckey 2003; Schollnberger et al. 2004; Feinendegen 2005).

Longevity is an important parameter for the health benefits of low-dose irradiation (Cameron 2003). A number of animal model studies have assessed the capacity of long-term whole body gamma rays to affect life span. The decrease of longevity in experimental animals is one of the well-known effects of high doses of ionizing radiation (Lamb 1964; Brown 1966; Giess and Planel 1977; Gould and Clark 1977; Giess 1980). However, enhanced longevity has been repeatedly found in lightly irradiated invertebrates and experimental animals. In all these experiments the mean life span was enhanced by 10–30% but not the maximum life span potential (Calabrese and Baldwin 2000). In this section, main focus is on the low-level radiation-induced mortality and life span modulation in both animal models and in epidemiological studies.

A number of reports describing the effects of the low-level irradiation are written in French and Russian, therefore they are largely unfamiliar to the English reader. In this review, the attempt is undertaken to fill this information gap.

Plant Growth Stimulation

Many reports discuss plant growth stimulation by exposure of plants to low doses of ionizing radiation (for review see Miller and Miller 1987). The reported effects include increased height, weight, growth rate, flowering and yield. The magnitude of the effects is usually small, being about 10% of control values; and these effects often are not reproducible. None has been independently confirmed. The exposure level reported to induce such effects is about one order of magnitude greater than that reported for similar hormetic responses in animals. There is no understanding of the exact mechanisms of such responses. Irradiation of seeds before planting can stimulate early plant growth, leading to advanced maturity and increased yield (Sheppard and Regitnig 1987). A hormetic response was observed for most species studied, but varied among cultivars and among seed lots within a cultivar. The response was most frequently evident at very early stages of growth and was often masked in subsequent growth. Seed condition may be the underlying factor in these effects. The unreliability of this response has limited its application. However, the technique has been extensively studied and now is practiced on a large scale by many farms in certain countries.

Invertebrate Studies

Nematode

Some controversial data were obtained concerning the effects of low dose irradiation on the survivorship and longevity of the nematode *Caenorhabditis elegans*. Pretreatment with ultraviolet or ionizing radiation did not promote subsequent resistance or increased longevity of the worms unlike multiple other stressors, including heat as well as pretreatment with hyperbaric oxygen or juglone (a chemical that generates reactive oxygen species) (Cypser and Johnson 2002). There was also a report of lack of lifespan extension in *C. elegans* after gamma-irradiation of dauer larvae (Yeargers 1981). On the other hand, occasional statistically significant but non-repeatable increases in survival of *C. elegans* were observed after intermediate levels of irradiation (10–30 krads) (Johnson and Hartman 1988). The radiation-sensitive mutants were about as sensitive as wild-type to the effects of ionizing radiation including occasional moderate life span extensions at intermediate doses.

Flour Beetle

The experiments of Davey (1917, 1919) with the flour beetle, *Tribolium confusum*, are one of the first studies presenting evidence consistent with the radiation hormetic hypothesis. In the daily exposure experiment of Davey (1917), five low doses of X-rays were applied [i.e., 100–500 mA/min at 25 cm at 50 kV (100–500 MAM/25^2 at 50 kV)] (cited in Calabrese and Baldwin 2000). The results of this experiment performed using 1,100 beetles in total indicated that the minimum dose needed to kill all the beetles was 500 MAM/25^2 at 50 kV, but the survival curves for 100 and 200 MAM/25^2 at 50 kV displayed a death rate lower than that observed in the controls. In the follow-up study of Davey (1919), the effects of X-rays on lifespan were assessed following either a single dose as in the Davey's (1917) study or via low daily X-ray exposures. In the daily exposure experiment, five doses were employed ranging from 6.25 to 50 MAM/25^2 at 50 kV daily with approximately 950 beetles per group. After 5 months nearly all the beetles had died. The mortality rates indicated that the three lowest irradiated groups displayed a 25–40% decrease in mortality by 30 days after the start of the study. The second experiment using about 850 beetles/group utilized a single dose in the range 100–400 MAM/25² at 50 kV. As in the earlier experiments, the lowest exposed groups again displayed a reduced mortality rate by 20 days after irradiation. According to Davey, the 1919 experiments provide a "direct confirmation" of his previous paper. He referred to the daily X-ray exposure as "a series of small 'homeopathic' doses", thereby linking the hormetic findings of his work to the medical practice of homeopathy. Forty years after Davey's experiments, Cork (1957) confirmed the life extending response in the same animal model, but using a gamma ray source (cesium-137) for either single or chronic daily doses. As in the case of Davey (1917, 1919), Cork likewise reported a marked extension of the lifespan in a well-designed study with large numbers of beetles.

Two decades later, Ducoff (1975) found that irradiation markedly increased life expectancy in sexually segregated *T. castaneum* adults of both sexes. Irradiation primarily reduced early mortality, making the survivorship curves more rectangular. However, there was little or no increase in maximum life span. Therefore, the author did not perceive this effect as necessarily beneficial, and so avoided 'the hormesis controversy' (Ducoff 1975). Further, he has postulated that the DNA damages which occurred during replication maintain repair activity at a genetically determined high level, but that repair capability would decline over time in terminally differentiated tissues. Accumulated lesions would interfere with gene transcription and, therefore, with adaptation to stresses. Thus, in mammals and other organisms highly dependent on cell proliferation, even low radiation doses would primarily be detrimental. By contrast, in organisms like insects, composed primarily of post-mitotic cells, radiation-induced increases in repair capability would lead to benefits from retardation of age-related decline in the ability to adapt to stress. The advantage of this concept was that it might be tested experimentally: if one could identify some stressors to which resistance declines with age, radiation exposure of young adults should retard this age-related decline. In checking this hypothesis, Lee and Ducoff (1983) did find that adult flour beetles became steadily more sensitive to hyperbaric oxygen and to heat, and that beetles which had been irradiated were more resistant to these stresses (Lee and Ducoff 1984; Ducoff and Lee 1984). However, stress resistance in the irradiated beetles was even considerably greater than in the young controls, so the effect was not simply a retardation of aging.

Housefly

Allen and Sohal (1982) have observed that low doses of gamma-irradiation enhance mean life span in the housefly, *Musca domestica*. In their study, adult houseflies of both sexes, exposed to 0, 20, 40 and 66 kR of gamma-radiation, were housed under conditions of relatively high or low physical activity. Under conditions of high activity, the mean life span of flies exposed to 20 and 40 kR was greater than in the controls, whereas the mean life span of all female populations, low activity males, and high activity males exposed to 66 kR was significantly decreased following irradiation.

Radiation exposure caused a reduction in the rate of oxygen consumption in both sexes. They reported that environmental conditions influence the longevity of male houseflies differently after an exposure to low dose of irradiation. The increased longevity is observed only when animals are reared in groups (promoting a high locomotor activity according to the authors). If singly reared (promoting a low locomotor activity), flies do not have higher longevities. Furthermore, irradiated flies have a higher longevity than controls only when these latter are kept in suboptimal rearing conditions. Radiation decreased the rate of fluorescent age pigment accumulation in high activity groups, but increased the rate of fluorescent age pigment accumulation under low activity conditions (Allen 1985). The authors suggested that radiation-induced life-lengthening in the housefly is a consequence of reduced metabolic activity (Allen and Sohal 1982).

Fruit Fly

The ionizing irradiation is widespread in fruit fly *Drosophila* studies. High doses of ionizing radiation are well known to cause life shortening of flies (Lamb 1964; Nelson 1973; Giess and Planel 1977; Gould and Clark 1977; Giess 1980). Dose fractionation resulted in a 'sparing' effect in adult male and female *D. melanogaster*; 24-, 48-, 72-, and 96-h-old females showed a higher recovery (increase in life span) following dose fractionation as compared to males of the respective age. Recovery in 72-h-old females was maximal (31% increase in life span) as against only 12% increase in the life span of the males (Mohsin 1979).

Low doses of gamma radiation were repeatedly shown to enhance the life span in *Drosophila* (Sacher 1963; Lamb 1964; Zainullin and Moskalev 2001; Moskalev et al. 2006; Vaiserman et al. 2003a, b, 2004). Sacher (1963), reporting increased longevity in irradiated *D. melanogaster*, had noted a reduction in variability of mean survival time between replicates of the irradiated samples, and he attributed both the reduction of variability and the improved survival to a reduction in the effectiveness of a deleterious environmental variable. By his point of view, 'it cannot be determined whether this reduced effectiveness results from an inactivation of the environmental factor or from an increase in resistance induced in the flies by the radiation exposure.' Lamb (1964) has assumed that irradiation leads to female sterility and that the longevity increase could be linked to a lower level of synthetic metabolism of the gonads. Supporting her hypothesis, she has shown that mutant females without ovaries do not exhibit a higher longevity after irradiation. Giess et al. (1980), on the contrary, postulated that radio-induced sterility is not accompanied by an alteration of the life expectancy: a 10kR dose which totally inhibits fertility and fertilizing power had no effect on the fruit fly lifespan. Thus, it causes doubt that the reduction in fecundity postulated by Lamb may be a plausible mechanism of the action of irradiation.

The role of programmed cell death (apoptosis) in radiation-induced lifespan modulation in *D. melanogaster* has been studied in the Komi Science Center (Syktyvkar, Russia). Chronic irradiation (accumulated doses between 0.6 and

0.8 Gy) was shown to change the life span in male *D. melanogaster*: mean life span was increased in wild-type strains and decreased in mutant strains defective in DNA repair and displaying a higher sensitivity to apoptosis induction (Zainullin and Moskalev 2001). In a *Drosophila* strain with dysfunction of the proapoptosis gene 'reaper' (rpr), an increase of life span was observed after irradiation and/or treatment with the apoptosis inductor etoposide (Moskalev and Zainullin 2001). Later, a relationship was observed between radio-induced apoptosis in larval ganglion cells and aging in *D. melanogaster* (Moskalev and Zainullin 2004) and a mechanism to explain the effect of low-dose irradiation on life span was proposed (Moskalev et al. 2006). The authors suggest that elimination of damaged or unwanted cells by the induction of apoptosis might slow aging and extend life span.

In our research conducted in the Kiev institute of gerontology, the effects of early-life X-ray irradiations were studied. The main objective of our investigations was to examine whether early-life low-level irradiations might cause 'epigenetic adaptation' in the treated fruit flies. An example of such kind of adaptation is epigenetic temperature adaptation in the birds, which can be easily achieved by changes in incubation temperature during the critical developmental phase. It has been shown, e.g., that prenatal temperature experiences induce post-natal warm or cold adaptation (Tzschentke et al. 2001; Loh et al. 2004; Tzschentke and Plagemann 2006). In one of our studies, the long-term consequences of the X-irradiation of fruit fly 1-h eggs with doses of 0.25, 0.50, 0.75, 1, 2 and 4 Gy were investigated (Vaiserman et al. 2003a). Longevity hormesis was observed in males exposed to 0.5 and 0.75 Gy, but no longevity increase was observed in females. Ultrastructural changes induced at the egg stage by irradiation at the dose of 0.75 Gy testified the increased transcriptional activity of the brain cells (Vaiserman et al. 2003b). The electrophoretic analysis has shown that the amount of the DNA segments resulting from cleavage in S1 nuclease-sensitive sites (<3 kb) reached 39.2% of the total DNA from control males. DNA from the irradiated males had a smaller amount of such fragments (10–30% in different experimental groups) (Fig. 1).

The higher stability of DNA originated from the irradiated flies could be the result of the activation of a repair system. In the light of these findings we concluded that the structural and/or functional DNA modifications, arising owing to irradiation at the egg stage, can persist in differentiated imaginal tissues. These modifications could alter the processes of repair and/or transcription, thus influencing adult life span. Also, it has been established that the effects of early-life X-irradiation may persist in subsequent generations. Following irradiation with 0.25, 0.5 and 0.75 Gy of 1-h eggs, both F0 and F1 flies showed a similar pattern of changes: they have decreased adult body weight and increased locomotor (photo- and geotactic) activity, whereas metabolic rate, measured as the rate of CO_2 production, was unchanged or even increased, and female fecundity was slightly reduced compared to appropriate controls. In some cases, irradiation resulted in hormetic effects: increased resistance to both starvation and heat shock stresses as well as life extension. An explanation of the beneficial long-lasting effects has been proposed, which suggests that these effects are due to irradiation-induced cross-life stage and cross-generational adaptive phenotypic plasticity (Vaiserman et al. 2004).

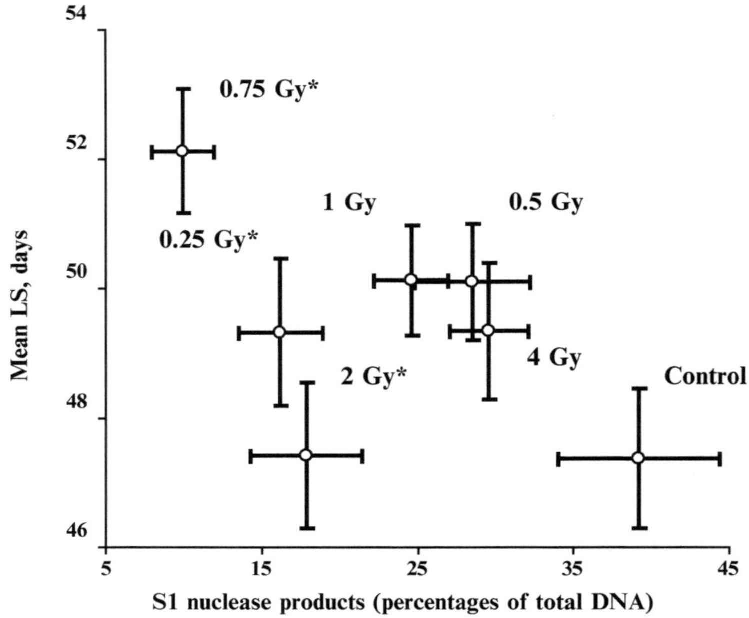

Fig. 1 Effect of irradiation with different doses at the egg stage on mean life span (LS) and percentages of the S1 nuclease products of *D. melanogaster* males. Standard errors are shown for estimates of both variables. Doses that produced significant increases in S1 nuclease products are marked with asterics (From Vaiserman et al. 2003a)

Rodent Studies

Starting in the early 1940s, Lorenz and his collaborators at the National Cancer Institute began an extended study of chronic low-level ionizing radiation effects in rodents. Lorenz et al. (1954) exposed groups of LAF_1 mice, guinea pigs, and rabbits to radium gamma rays for 8 h/day, beginning at young adult age and continuing until all were dead. The levels of daily dose given were 8.8, 4.4, 2.2, 1.1, and 0.11 R/day. The exposed animals had longer life spans by 2–14% and 50% greater body weight than unexposed ones. Increased tumor incidence was also observed at the 0.11 R level in mice. These findings were confirmed in a later study (Lorenz et al. 1955). The primary hypothesis for increased median life span has been rebound regenerative hyperplasia during the early part of the exposure; in the presence of continuing injury, there is physiological enhancement of defence mechanisms against intercurrent infection. Later, Carlson and co-workers (Carlson et al. 1957; Carlson and Jackson 1959), studying the combined effects of ionizing radiation and heat or cold, gave gamma irradiation to rats for 12 months at daily doses ranging from 0.3 to 4.0 R/day. An increase of median and maximum survival time above control values was observed in the exposed groups over this entire dose range, with a significant peak increase of 30% at 2.5 R/day.

More recently, chronic gamma irradiation at very low-dose rates of 7 or 14 cGy/year was shown to significantly extend the life span of female C57BL/6 mice: median survival time was 549 days in controls and 673 days in both irradiated groups (Caratero et al. 1998). However, in a subsequent study (Courtade et al. 2002), no statistical differences in life span as well as in cancer or non-cancer diseases were detected between irradiated and non-irradiated mice. Chronic low-dose-rate γ irradiation at 0.35 or 1.2 mGy/h prolonged the life span of MRL-lpr/lpr mice carrying a deletion in the apoptosis-regulating *Fas* gene that markedly shortens life due to severe autoimmune disease (Ina and Sakai 2004). The extension of the irradiation period to the entire life of the mice at the same dose rates improved survival further (Ina and Sakai 2005). The 50% survival time for untreated mice, 134 days, was prolonged to 502 days by 1.2 mGy/h lifelong irradiation. Activation of the immune system was obtained, as indicated by a significant increase in CD4+ CD8+ T cells in the thymus and CD8+ T cells in the spleen and also by a significant decrease in CD3+ CD45R/B220+ cells and CD45R/B220+ CD40+ cells in the spleen. However, no evidence of lengthened life span in mice continuously exposed to very low dose rates of γ rays was shown by Tanaka et al. (2003). Using a total of 4,000 mice, they studied the late biological effects of chronic exposure to low-dose-rate radiation as assayed by life span. Irradiation was carried out for approximately 400 days using ^{137}Cs γ rays at dose rates of 21, 1.1 and 0.05 mGy/day with total doses equivalent to 8,000, 400 and 20 mGy, respectively. The life spans of mice of both sexes irradiated with 21 mGy and of females irradiated with 1.1 mGy/day were significantly shorter than those of the control group.

The radiation hormesis was also obtained in the chipmunk, *Tamias striatus* (Thompson et al. 1990). Wild chipmunks were captured, exposed to single doses of either 200 or 400 rad ionizing radiation, and subsequently returned to their natural habitat. The irradiated chipmunks exhibited a biphasic response in age-specific mortality rate. A residuum of unrepaired toxicity (injury) appeared to persist and manifest itself throughout life. A second response, longevity hormesis, was also observed.

Detrimental Effects of Suppressing Background Radiation

Numerous facts indicating that background ionizing radiation may be essential for life provided a strong argument in favor of a beneficial effect of low level radiation. This might be expected because life on Earth has evolved under constant exposure to ionizing radiation, which 3.5 billion years ago was about three times higher than now (Jaworowski 1997).

Indeed, exposure to lower than natural radiation has been shown to cause deficiency symptoms in protozoa and bacteria. A group of studies carried out by Planel and his associates at the University of Toulouse as early as in the 1960s indicate that protozoa and bacteria exposed to artificially lowered levels of natural radiation demonstrate deficiency symptoms expressed as dramatically decreased proliferation (Planel et al. 1966, 1969). In a later research, the blue-green alga, *Synechococcus lividus*, was grown under various levels of radiations. Shielding of cultures with lead resulted in a lower cell growth rate: the reduction disappeared when a normal radiation level was restored in the lead chamber. Irradiations from a thorium source at a dose-rate 14 times higher than that of natural irradiation stimulated the growth of the algae (Conter et al. 1983). A more recent study carried out on the protozoan *Paramecium tetraurelia* and the cyanobacteria *Synechococcus lividus*, which were shielded against background radiation or exposed to very low doses of gamma radiation, demonstrated that radiation can stimulate the proliferation of these two single-cell organisms.

In the Planel et al.'s study (1987), the protozoan *Paramecium tetraurelia* and the cyanobacteria *Synechococcus lividus* were shielded against background radiation or exposed to very low doses of gamma radiation: this study demonstrated that radiation can stimulate the proliferation of these two single-cell organisms (Fig. 2). Radiation hormesis depends on internal factors (age of starting cells) and external factors (lighting conditions). The stimulatory effect occurred only in a limited range of doses and disappeared for dose rates higher than 50 mGy/year.

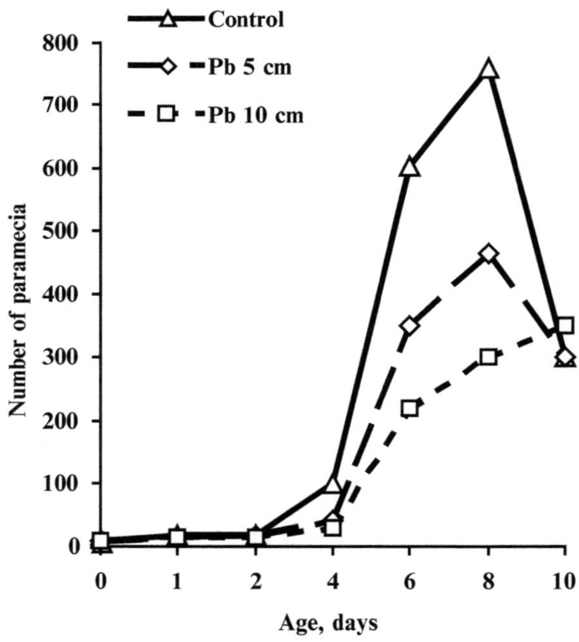

Fig. 2 Effect of shielding on proliferation of *Paramecium tetraurelia* cultured in identical chambers which were shielded from background radiation with either 5 or 10 cm of lead (From Planel et al. 1987)

Similar results were obtained with *D. melanogaster*. It has been shown that protecting from natural ionizing radiation delayed development of fruit flies (Planel et al. 1967a), decreased reproductive performance (Planel et al. 1967b) and life span (Giess and Planel 1973; Planel and Giess 1973). In the last study, two populations of *D. melanogaster* were compared. The control group experienced the normal ambient radiation exposure, while the experimental group, from egg to death, experienced 10% of the natural gamma ray background irradiation. The outcome (five trials for each sex, involving a total of 10,000 flies) was a decrease of average survival time from 9.73 weeks for controls to 9.01 weeks in the shielded group, a difference of 7.4% (Planel and Giess 1973).

Overall, these data suggest a role of background ionizing radiation in determining of adaptive features. Basing on this data, Sacher (1977) has assumed that 'organisms might depend on the statistically uniform level of free radicals produced by background radiation as primers for certain metabolic reactions.'

Epidemiological Studies

Study of Radiologist's Mortality

Radiologists and radiotherapists were one of the earliest occupational groups to be exposed to ionizing radiation. The mortality experience of radiologists compared to that of other physician specialists demonstrates an increased risk of cancer deaths as well as deaths from all causes among physicians practicing in the early years of 20th century. However, for the radiologists who joined specialty societies after 1940, the age pattern of deaths has changed (Matanoski et al. 1987). Whereas among early entrants, young radiologists had higher mortality rates than those of other specialists, among later entrants, the young radiologists have lower mortality. However, as these later-entrant radiologists age, their rates appear to exceed those of other specialists. In a paper on the mortality of British radiologists over the 100 years from 1897 to 1997, Berrington et al. (2001) reported that the mortality of those who had registered since 1954 was remarkably low in comparison with that of medical practitioners as a whole. This was true both for cancer and for all other causes of death combined. In discussing this paper, Cameron (2002) stressed that 'the British radiology data show that moderate doses of radiation are beneficial rather than a risk to health.' But later it has been concluded that the low mortality of British radiologists who were registered in the period 1955–1997, in comparison with that for all medical practitioners, is attributable to the factors that cause a relatively low mortality in doctors in all medical specialties; therefore, there is no reason to attribute it to a specific benefit from exposure to low doses of ionizing radiation (Doll et al. 2005). Yoshinaga et al. (2004) reviewed epidemiologic data on cancer risks from eight cohorts of over 270,000 radiologists and technologists in various countries.

The most consistent finding was increased mortality due to leukemia among early workers employed before 1950, when radiation exposures were high. This, together with an increasing risk of leukemia with increasing duration of work in the early years, provided evidence of an excess risk of leukemia associated with occupational radiation exposure in that period. However, there is no clear evidence of an increased cancer risk in medical radiation workers exposed to current levels of radiation doses.

A-Bomb Survivors Study

A-bomb survivors studies generally indicate that acute irradiation with absorbed doses of more than about 0.1–0.2 Gy/person increases cancer risk in the exposed groups proportionally with dose up to about 2 Gy (Pierce et al. 1996; Pierce and Preston 2000). However, no evidence for risk increase after absorbed doses below 0.1 Gy was obtained (Heidenreich et al. 1997; Preston et al. 2004). Shimizu et al. (1999) have published the results of the updated analysis of deaths from causes other than cancer among the Japanese survivors of the atomic bomb explosions, covering the period 1950–1990. The primary analyses are based on 27,000 deaths. These findings confirm a statistically significant trend of an increasing rate of non-cancer mortality with increasing dose, due to trends for diseases of circulatory, digestive and respiratory systems. At 1 Sv, the proportional increase is about 10%, much smaller than for cancer (at around 50%), but the numbers of excess deaths are more comparable. The authors concluded that the question of dose–response relationship remains unresolved: linearity is possible, but the data are also consistent with a threshold at 0.5 Sv. In contrast, there is evidence for protective effect of low doses of irradiation on cancer development. According to Mine et al. (1990), among about 100,000 A-bomb survivors registered at Nagasaki University School of Medicine, 290 male subjects exposed to 50–149 cGy showed significantly lower mortality from non-cancerous diseases than age-matched unexposed males. According to UNSCEAR report (1994), among A-bomb survivors from Hiroshima and Nagasaki who received doses lower than 200 mSv, there was no increase in the number of deaths due to cancers. Mortality caused by leukemia was even lower in this population at doses below 100 mSv than in age-matched control cohorts. However, Cologne and Preston (2000) results do not support claims that survivors exposed to low or moderate doses of radiation live longer than comparable unexposed individuals. In their study, among atomic bomb survivors, the mean life expectancy for city residents who were not in the city at the time of the explosion was 81 years 155 days, while the mean life expectancy for survivors with doses in the range of 5–250 mGy (mean, 60 mGy) was 81 years 9 days. In addition, it has been shown that participation in United Kingdom's atmospheric nuclear weapon tests had no detectable effect on expectation of life or on subsequent risk of developing cancer or other fatal diseases (Darby et al. 1993).

Nuclear Workers Study

Cardis et al. (2005), in their studies of 407,391 nuclear plant workers in 15 countries, concluded that 1–2% of cancer deaths among the cohort may be due to radiation. In a cohort study of mortality among 954 Canadian military personnel exposed to low-dose ionizing radiation during nuclear reactor clean-up operations in Chalk River, Ontario, no elevation in the frequency of death from leukemia or thyroid cancer was found in the exposed groups (Raman et al. 1987). Analysis of survival by recorded gamma radiation dose also did not show any effect of radiation dose on mortality. Canadian studies examining the effect of occupational radiation exposure among nuclear industry workers found that cancer mortality in this population was 58% of the national average (Abbatt et al. 1983). In United Kingdom, a negative association was found between radiation exposure and mortality from cancer, in particular leukemia (excluding chronic lymphatic leukemia) and multiple myeloma (Kendall et al. 1992). Matanoski (1993) studied workers of US nuclear shipyards. Significantly lower standardized mortality rates were reported in workers overhauling nuclear-powered ships with cumulative effective doses greater than 5 mSv than in those with lower doses, and in the latter group compared with non-radiation shipyard workers. However, the author of the study did not suggest that these results provide evidence for a beneficial effect of radiation but instead regarded selection bias as a more likely cause.

Background Radiation Study

Many studies examining health effects of background radiation have reported that populations in areas with high-background radiation rates show no adverse health effects when compared to low-dose populations. Several studies of large populations with significant differences in doses indicate beneficial health effects, i.e., lower mortality and disease rates. A Chinese study compared an area with average radiation exposure of 2.31 mSv/year with a similar area with 0.96 mSv/year average exposure (High Background Radiation Research Group 1980). The cancer mortality rate was lower in the high-background group, but this difference was statistically significant only in the 40- to 70-years age group (i.e., those who had the greatest lifelong exposure to high background levels of radiation). In a large-scale Chinese study of the residents of high background radiation area, the cancer mortality rate was lower in the area with a relatively high background radiation (74,000 people), while the control group who lived in an area with low background radiation (78,000 people) had a higher rate of mortality (Wei et al. 1990). In a similar Indian study, the cancer incidence/mortality rates was significantly less in areas with a high-background radiation level than in similar areas with a low background radiation level (Nambi and Soman 1987). A lower cancer mortality was reported among inhabitants in the Misasa spa area (Japan), where there is a high radon background, than in the whole Japanese population (Mifune et al. 1992). Cohen (1993) found a significant negative correlation between average radon levels and mortality rates from the lung cancer in 1,600 US counties. The comparison of three Rocky Mountain States (Idaho, Colorado, New Mexico) with three Gulf States (Louisiana, Mississippi, Alabama) in the USA showed a strong negative correlation between natural radon levels and estimated lung cancer mortality (Jagger 1998). In a very large scale study in the USA, the mortality rate due to all malignancies was lower in states with higher annual radiation dose (Frigerio 1976).

In the majority of recent reviews, attention was drawn to results that demonstrate health benefits of low-dose ionizing radiation. Summarizing these points, Cameron (2005) stated that 'we need increased background radiation to improve our health.' However, as Brenner and Hall (2003) point out, estimation of the effects of radiation on a human population receiving annual occupational doses of less than 1 mGy is extraordinarily difficult, because the standard mortality ratios are close to unity. In such a situation, most studies would be expected to show no statistically significant effects; occasionally one study will show an effect in one direction and another will show an effect in the other direction. Therefore, it is important to look carefully at all the available evidence before reaching a conclusion that a low dose of X-rays increases longevity (Brenner and Hall 2003; Hall and Brenner 2003).

Can Low-Level Radiation Cause Harm?

There is increasing evidence that both radiation-induced genomic instability and bystander effects play a role in low dose radiation responses. The bystander effect refers to the induction of biological effects in cells that are not directly traversed by a charged particle (Hall 2003). Irradiated cells induce chromosomal instability in unirradiated bystander cells in vitro. For example, in cell cultures irradiated so that only 1% of the cells sustained a collision with an α-particle, sister chromatid exchanges were observed in >30% of the cells (Nagasawa and Little 1992). Other studies have also supported this model (for review see, e.g., Zhou et al. 2001). These effects suggest that irradiated cells may signal their distress to other cells, perhaps by direct cell-to-cell interaction or by molecules secreted into the medium. The latter form of cellular communication is supported by findings showing that the bystander effect could be induced in non-irradiated cell cultures incubated with conditioned medium from irradiated cultures (Mothersill and Seymour 1998). There is evidence that bystander effects do occur in vivo (Brooks 2004; Koturbash et al. 2006). The contribution of bystander effects in vivo may significantly alter biological responses to low dose radiation exposure and could result in a cancer-protective effect by eliminating genetically compromised cells or low dose hypersensitivity. If a bystander effect is indeed induced in vivo after chronic exposure to low dose radiation, this would challenge the assumed linearity of low radiation dose effects and suggest a possible mechanism for previously observed hormetic and hypersensitive low dose responses. Opposite to the adaptive response model, the bystander-effect model postulates that low-dose radiation may be even more damaging than that predicted by the linear non-threshold model (for reviews see, e.g., Bonner 2003; Prise et al. 2003).

Recently, it has been recognized that ionizing radiation not only increases mutation rates in the exposed somatic cells but also results in an elevated mutation rate in many cell divisions after the initial irradiation damage (Morgan et al. 1996; Barber et al. 2002). If genomic instability is also induced in the germ line of exposed parents then delayed transgenerational effects may be manifested in their offspring, therefore presenting greater delayed risk in populations exposed to ionizing radiation. In the early studies of radiation-induced genomic instability, it was usually assumed that low-dose rate of chronic gamma-irradiation does not likely cause any risk of damaging effects to the offspring of the irradiated animals. For example, Luke et al. (1997) found that pre-conceptional paternal exposure to 0.1 Gy gamma-rays did not increase any risk, and even decreased mutations (genomic instability) in F1 offspring mice, but exposure to 1–4 Gy caused a markedly increased effect. This suggested that the dose <0.2 Gy should not significantly increase the risk for the genomic alteration in the offspring of paternally exposed individuals. In the Cai and Wang's study (1995), a very low-dose rate (20 microGy/min) of chronic ^{60}Co gamma-irradiation was used to pre-irradiate mice for 40 days. Then, 40 days later, these mice were treated with a subsequent large dose of X-irradiation, followed 24 h later by cytogenetic analysis of their spermatocytes. Analysis for radiation-induced DNA and chromosomal damage was also carried out in splenocytes, bone marrow cells and spermatocytes of the offspring of mice adapted by the low-dose rate of chronic gamma-irradiation. Results demonstrated that (i) cumulative gamma-irradiation (1.10 Gy) at the dose rate 20 microGy/min induced a marked cytogenetic adaptive response in the mouse germ cells (stem spermatogonia); (ii) the sensitivity of offspring's bone marrow cells and spermatocytes to 1.5 Gy X-ray-induced chromosome aberrations was not influenced by the low-dose radiation delivered to paternal germ cells; (iii) either constitutive or post-irradiation DNA repair capacity (UV-induced unscheduled DNA synthesis) was not modified in the offspring's splenocytes; (iv) the sensitivity of the offspring's splenocytes to radiation-induced cell killing was also not altered. These results suggest that low-dose radiation delivered to the male parents with a significant induction of cytogenetic adaptive response in their germ cell does not likely cause any risk of damaging effects to the offspring of those irradiated male mice. Iwasaki et al. (1996) observed a very low incidence of heritable effects in the offspring of paternal exposure to low- or moderate-level radiation. C57BL/6 male mice were exposed to 3 Gy ^{60}Co gamma-rays and mated with unirradiated females after 15 days to produce F1 progeny. After weaning the offspring were allowed to live their normal life span. No significant differences in the survival curve and mean life span between the irradiated and control groups were noted. The only radiation effect in tumor incidence was a decrease of histiocytic sarcoma in female offspring of irradiated males. Except for this, there were no significant differences between the irradiated group and the control group in the incidence or age distribution of tumors. This may be due to the efficiently selective elimination of cells with genomic abnormality probably by apoptotic cell death.

However, it has recently been shown that low-dose chronic exposure to ionizing radiation could be substantially more mutagenic than previously thought. A number of studies on mice have reported elevated mutation rates in the germ line of the low-dose irradiated animals. The mutation rates at tandem repeat DNA loci and protein-coding genes in the offspring of irradiated males was substantially elevated across multiple tissues (Dubrova et al. 2000; Barber et al. 2002, 2006). Mutation rates at two expanded simple tandem repeat loci were, e.g., studied in the germ line of first- and second-generation offspring of inbred male CBA/H, C57BL/6, and BALB/c mice exposed to either high linear energy transfer fission neutrons or low linear energy transfer X-rays (Barber et al. 2002). Paternal CBA/H exposure to either X-rays or fission neutrons resulted in increased mutation rates in the germ line of two subsequent generations. Comparable transgenerational effects were observed also in neutron-irradiated C57BL/6 and X-irradiated BALB/c mice. The remarkable transgenerational destabilisation is attributed to the presence of a persistent subset of DNA lesions, such as double- and single-strand breaks (Barber et al. 2006). It has been shown that the doubling dose for germ line mutation induction at mouse minisatellite loci by acute irradiation with X-rays was 0.33 Gy (Dubrova et al. 1998). Zanchkina et al. (2002) studied the genomic instability in somatic cells of the progeny (F1 generation) of male mice chronically exposed to low-dose gamma-radiation by comparative analysis of chromosome damage. BALB/C male mice exposed to 0.1 Gy (0.01 Gy/day) and 0.5 Gy (0.01 and 0.05 Gy/day) were mated with unirradiated females 15 days after irradiation: a gamma-radiation-induced genomic instability was detected in both parental germ cells and F1 offspring somatic cells.

Thus the question of whether low levels of radiation can cause harm remains controversial. The possibility of potential harm makes it difficult to use low-level irradiation as a therapeutic tool at present. It is generally felt that more in-depth studies of its possible negative effects should be undertaken.

References

Abbatt JD, Hamilton TR and Weeks JL (1983) Epidemiological studies in three corporations covering the Canadian nuclear fuel cycle. In: Biological Effects of Low-Level Radiation, pp. 351–361. IAEA Symposium Proceedings, Vienna, Austria

Allen RG (1985) Relationship between gamma-irradiation, life span, metabolic rate and accumulati on of fluorescent age pigment in the adult male housefly, *Musca domestica*. Arch Gerontol Geriatr 4: 169–178

Allen RG and Sohal RS (1982) Life-lengthening effects of gamma-radiation on the adult housefly, *Musca domestica*. Mech Ageing Dev 20: 369–375

Atkinson GF (1898) Report upon some preliminary experiments with Roentgen rays on plants. Science 7: 7

Barber C, Hickenbotham P, Hatch T and Kelly D (2006) Radiation-induced transgenerational alterations in genome stability and DNA damage. Oncogene 25: 7336–7342

Barber R, Plumb MA, Boulton E, Roux I and Dubrova YE (2002) Elevated mutation rates in the germline of first- and second-generation offspring of irradiated male mice. Proc Natl Acad Sci USA 99: 6877–6882

Berrington A, Darby SC, Weiss HA and Doll R (2001) 100 years of observation on British radiologists: mortality from cancer and other causes 1897–1997. Br J Radiol 74: 507–519

Bonner WM (2003) Low-dose radiation: thresholds, bystander effects, and adaptive responses. Proc Natl Acad Sci USA 100: 4973–4975

Brenner DJ and Hall EJ (2003) Mortality patterns in British and US radiologists: what can we really conclude? Br J Radiol 76: 1–2

Brooks AL (2004) Evidence for 'bystander effects' in vivo. Hum Exp Toxicol 23: 67–70

Brown B (1966) Long-term radiation damage evaluation of life–span studies. Memorandum. RM–5083–TAB. The Rand Corporation, Santa Monica, CA

Brucer M (1990) A Chronology of Nuclear Medicine, Heritage Publications, St. Louis

Cai L and Wang P (1995) Induction of a cytogenetic adaptive response in germ cells of irradiated mice with very low-dose rate of chronic gamma-irradiation and its biological influence on radiation-induced DNA or chromosomal damage and cell killing in their male offspring. Mutagenesis 10: 95–100

Calabrese EJ and Baldwin LA (2000) Radiation hormesis: its historical foundations as a biological hypothesis. Hum Exp Toxicol 19: 41–75

Calabrese EJ and Baldwin LA (2000) The effects of gamma rays on longevity. Biogerontology 1: 309–319

Cameron JR (2002) Radiation increased the longevity of British radiologists. Br J Radiol 75: 637–639

Cameron JR (2003) Longevity is the most appropriate measure of health effects of radiation. Radiology 229: 13–14

Cameron JR (2005) Moderate dose rate ionizing radiation increases longevity. Br J Radiol 78: 11–13

Caratero A, Courtade M, Bonnet L, Planel H and Caratero C (1998) Effect of a continuous gamma irradiation at a very low dose on the life span of mice. Gerontology 44: 272–276

Cardis E, Vrijheld M, Blettner M, Gilbert E, Hakama M, Hill C et al. (2005) Risk of cancer after low doses of ionising radiation: retrospective cohort study in 15 countries. BMJ 2005 331: 77–80

Carlson LD and Jackson BH (1959) The combined effects of ionizing radiation and high temperature on the longevity of the Sprague–Dawley rat. Radiat Res 11: 509–519

Carlson LD, Scheyer WJ and Jackson BH (1957) The combined effects of ionizing radiation and low temperature on the metabolism, longevity and soft tissue of the white rat. Radiat Res 7: 190–195

Cohen BL (1993) Relationship between exposure to radon and various types of cancer. Health Phys 65: 529–531

Cologne JB and Preston DL (2000) Longevity of atomic–bomb survivors. Lancet 356: 303–307

Conter A, Dupouy D and Planel H (1983) Demonstration of a biological effect of natural ionizing radiation. Int J Rad Biol 43: 421–432

Cork JM (1957) Gamma–radiation and longevity of the flour beetle. Radiat Res 7: 551–557

Courtade M, Billote C, Gasset G, Caratero A, Charlet JP, Pipy B and Caratero C (2002) Life span, cancer and non-cancer diseases in mouse exposed to a continuous very low dose of gamma-irradiation. Int J Radiat Biol 78: 845–855

Cypser JR and Johnson TE (2002) Multiple stressors in *Caenorhabditis elegans* induce stress hormesis and extended longevity. J Gerontol Biol Sci 57: 109–114

Darby SC, Kendall GM, Fell TP, Doll R, Goodill AA, Conquest AJ, Jackson DA and Haylock RG (1993) Further follow up of mortality and incidence of cancer in men from the United Kingdom who participated in the United Kingdom's atmospheric nuclear weapon tests and experimental programmes. BMJ 307: 1530–1535

Davey WP (1917) The effect of X-rays on the length of life of *Tribolium confusum*. J Exp Zool 22: 573–592

Davey WP (1919) Prolongation of life of *Tribolium confusum* apparently due to small doses of X-rays. Journal of Experimental Zoology 28: 447–458

Doll R, Berrington A and Darby SC (2005) Low mortality of British radiologists Br J Radiol 78: 1057–1058
Dubrova YE, Plumb M, Brown J, Fennelly J, Bois P, Goodhead D and Jeffreys AJ (1998) Stage specificity, dose response, and doubling dose for mouse minisatellite germ-line mutation induced by acute radiation. Proc Natl Acad Sci USA 95: 6251–6255
Dubrova YE, Plumb M, Gutierrez B, Boulton E and Jeffreys AJ (2000). Transgenerational mutation by radiation. Nature 405: 37
Ducoff HS (1975) Form of the increased longevity of *Tribolium* after X-irradiation. Exp Gerontol 10: 189–193
Ducoff HS and Lee YJ (1984) Radiation-induced resistance to heat and to oxygen. In: Overgaard J (ed) Hyperthermic Oncology, pp. 297–300. Taylor & Francis, London
Feinendegen LE (2005) Evidence for beneficial low level radiation effects and radiation hormesis. Br J Radiol 78: 3–7
Frigerio NA and Stowe RS (1976) Carcinogenic and genetic hazard from background radiation. In: Biological and environmental effects of low-level radiation, pp. 385–393. IAEA Symposium Proceedings, Vol. II, Vienna, Austria
Giess MC (1980) Differences between natural ageing and radio-induced shortening of the life expectancy in *Drosophila melanogaster*. Gerontology 26: 301–310
Giess MC and Planel H (1973) Effect of radioprotection at different periods on the longevity of Drosophila melanogaster. C R Acad Sci Hebd Seances Acad Sci D 276: 1029–1032 [in French]
Giess MC and Planel H (1977) Influence of sex on the radiation-induced lifespan modifications in *Drosophila melanogaster*. Gerontology 23: 325–333
Giess MC, Cazeaux S and Murat M (1980) Post-radiative sterility and lifespan in males and females of *Drosophila melanogaster*. Exp Gerontol 15: 503–510
Gould AB and Clark AM (1977) X-ray induced mutations causing adult life-shorting in *Drosophila melanogaster*. Exp Gerontol 12: 107–112
Hall EJ (2003) The bystander effect. Health Phys 85: 31–35
Hall EJ and Brenner DJ (2003) The weight of evidence does not support the suggestion that exposure to low doses of X-rays increases longevity. Radiology 229: 18–19
Heidenreich WF, Paretzke HG and Jacob P (1997) No evidence for increased tumor rates below 200 mSv in the atomic bomb survivor data. Radiat Environ Biophys 36: 205–207
High Background Radiation Research Group (1980) Health survey in high background radiation areas in China. Science 209: 877–880
Hunter PE and Krithayakiern V (1971) Effect of gamma radiation upon life expectancy and reproduction in the house cricket, *Acheta domesticus* (*Orthoptera: Gryllidae*). Ann Entomol Soc Am 64: 119–123
Ina Y and Sakai K (2004) Prolongation of life span associated with immunological modification by chronic low-dose-rate irradiation in MRL–lpr/lpr mice. Radiat Res 161: 168–173
Ina Y and Sakai K (2005) Further study of prolongation of life span associated with immunological modification by chronic low-dose-rate irradiation in MRL–lpr/lpr mice: effects of whole-life irradiation. Radiat Res 163: 418–423
Iwasaki T, Hashimoto N, Endoh D, Imanisi T, Itakura C and Sato F (1996) Life span and tumors in the first-generation offspring of the gamma-irradiated male mouse. Int J Radiat Biol 69: 487–492
Jagger J (1998) Natural background radiation and cancer death in Rocky Mountain States and Gulf Coast States. Health Phys 75: 428–430
Jaworowski Z (1997) Radiation 3.5 billion years ago. 21st Century Sci Technol 10: 4
Johnson TE and Hartman PS (1988) Radiation effects on life span in *Caenorhabditis elegans*. J Gerontol 43: 137–141
Kendall GM, Muirhead CR, MacGibbon BH, O'Hagan JA, Conquest AJ, Goodill AA et al. (1992) Mortality and occupational exposure to radiation: first analysis of the National Registry for Radiation Workers. BMJ 304: 220–225
Koturbash I, Rugo RE, Hendricks CA, Loree J, Thibault B, Kutanzi K, Pogribny I, Yanch JC, Engelward BP and Kovalchuk O (2006) Irradiation induces DNA damage and modulates epigenetic effectors in distant bystander tissue *in vivo*. Oncogene 25: 4267–4275

Lamb MJ (1964) The effect of radiation on the longevity of female *Drosophila subobscura*. J Insect Physiol 10: 487–497
Lee YJ and Ducoff HS (1983) Age and sensitivity to oxygen in the flour beetle, *Tribolium confusum*. Mech Age Dev 22: 97–103
Lee YJ and Ducoff HS (1984) Radiation-enhanced resistance to oxygen: a possible relationship to radiation-enhanced longevity. Mech Age Dev 27: 101–109
Loh B, Maier I, Winar A, Janke O and Tzschentke B (2004) Prenatal development of epigenetic adaptation processes in poultry: changes in metabolic and neuronal thermoregulatory mechanisms. Avian Poult Biol Rev 15: 119–128
Lorenz E, Hollcroft JW, Miller E, Congdon CC and Schweisthal R (1955) Long-term effects of acute and chronic irradiation in mice. I. Survival and tumor incidence following chronic irradiation of 0.11 r per day. J Natl Cancer Inst 15: 1049–1058
Lorenz E, Jacobson LO, Heston EW, Shimkin M, Eschenbrenner AB, Deringer MK, Doniger J and Schweisthal R (1954) Effects of long-continued total-body gamma irradiation on mice, guinea pigs, and rabbits. III. Effects on life span, weight, blood picture, and carcinogenesis and the role of the intensity of radiation. In: Zirkle RE (ed) Biological Effects of X and Gamma Radiation, pp. 24–148. McGraw-Hill, New York
Luckey TD (1991) Radiation Hormesis. CRC, Boca Raton, FL
Luckey TD (1993) Radiation hormesis: biopositive effect of radiations. Plenary lecture presented at the 7th GIRI meeting, November 1993, Montpellier, France. Available from: http://www.giriweb.com/luckey.htm
Luckey TD (1999) Radiation hormesis overview. Radiat Prot Manage 16: 22–34
Luckey TD (2003) Radiation hormesis overview. RSO Magazine 8: 19–36
Luke GA, Riches AC and Bryant PE (1997) Genomic instability in hematopoietic cells of F1 generation mice of irradiated male parents. Mutagenesis 12: 147–152
Macklis RM (1990) Radithor and the era of mild radium therapy. JAMA 264: 614–618
Matanoski GM (1993) Nuclear shipyard workers study. Radiat Res 133: 126–127
Matanoski GM, Sternberg A and Elliott EA (1987) Does radiation exposure produce a protective effect among radiologists? Health Phys 52: 637–643
Mifune M, Sobue T, Arimoto H, Komoto Y, Kondo S and Tanooka H (1992) Cancer mortality survey in a spa area (Misasa, Japan) with a high radon background. Jpn J Cancer Res 83: 1–5
Miller MW and Miller WM (1987) Radiation hormesis in plants. Health Phys 52: 607–616
Mine M, Okumura Y, Ichimaru M, Nakamura T and Kondo S (1990) Apparently beneficial effect of low to intermediate doses of A–bomb radiation on human life span. Int J Radiat Biol 58: 1035–1043
Mohsin A (1979) The sparing effect of dose-fractionation in adult *Drosophila*. Experientia 35: 746–747
Morgan WF, Day JP, Kaplan MI, McGhee EM, Limoli CL (1996) Genomic instability induced by ionizing radiation. Radiat Res 146: 247–258
Moskalev AA and Zainullin VG (2001) Role of apoptotic cell death in radio induced aging in *Drosophila melanogaster*. Radiats Biol Radioecol 41: 650–652 [in Russian]
Moskalev AA and Zainullin VG (2004) Aging rate after continual low dose irradiation of *Drosophila* strains with apoptosis deregulation. Radiats Biol Radioecol 44: 156–161 [in Russian]
Moskalev AA, Iatskiv AS and Zainullin VG (2006) Effect of low-dose irradiation on the lifespan in various strains of *Drosophila melanogaster*. Genetika 42: 773–782 [in Russian]
Mothersill C and Seymour C (1998) Cell–cell contact during gamma irradiation is not required to induce a bystander effect in normal human keratinocytes: evidence for release during irradiation of a signal controlling survival into the medium. Radiat Res 149: 256–262
Nagasawa H and Little JB (1992) Induction of sister chromatid exchanges by extremely low doses of alpha-particles. Cancer Res 52: 6394–6396
Nambi KSV and Soman SD (1987) Environmental radiation and cancer in India. Health Phys 52: 653–657
Nelson FR (1973) *Drosophila melanogaster*: effects of gamma radiation on fecundity and longevity. J Econ Entomol 66: 257–258

Pierce DA and Preston DL (2000) Radiation-related cancer risks at low doses among atomic bomb survivors. Radiat Res 154: 178–186

Pierce DA, Shimizu Y, Preston DL, Vaeth M and Mabuchi K (1996) Studies of the mortality of atomic bomb survivors. Report 12, Part I: 1950–1990. Radiat Res 146: 1–27

Planel H and Giess MC (1973) Decrease in the longevity of Drosophila melanogaster caused by protection against natural ionizing radiations. C R Acad Sci Hebd Seances Acad Sci D 676: 809–812 [in French]

Planel H, Soleilhavoup JP, Blanc D, Fontan J and Tixador R (1966) Action of the gamma radiation of thorium on the growth of Paramecium caudatum and Paramecium aurelia grown under radioprotective apparatus. C R Acad Sci Hebd Seances Acad Sci D 160: 1090–1093 [in French]

Planel H, Soleilhavoup JP, Cottin F, Tixador R and Richoilley G (1969) Biologic action of natural irradiation: study of the growth of Paramecium aurelia and Paramecium caudatum in a subterranean laboratory. C R Acad Sci Hebd Seances Acad Sci D 269: 1697–1700 [in French]

Planel H, Soleilhavoup JP, Giess MC and Tixador R (1967a) Demonstration of a retardation of development of Drosophila melanogaster by diminution of environmental natural radioactivity. C R Acad Sci Hebd Seances Acad Sci D 264: 865–868 [in French]

Planel H, Soleilhavoup JP, Giess MC and Tixador R (1967b) Action of natural ionizing radiations on the reproduction of metazoa: studies on Drosophila. C R Acad Sci Hebd Seances Acad Sci D 264: 755–758 [in French]

Planel H, Soleilhavoup JP, Tixador R, Richoilley G, Conter A, Croute F, Caratero C and Gaubin Y (1987) Influence on cell proliferation of background radiation or exposure to very low, chronic gamma radiation. Health Phys 52: 571–578

Preston DL, Pierce DA, Shimizu Y, Cullings HM, Fujita S, Funamoto S and Kodama K (2004) Effect of recent changes in atomic bomb survivor dosimetry on cancer mortality risk estimates. Radiat Res 162: 377–389

Prise KM, Folkard M and Michael BD (2003) A review of the bystander effect and its implications for low–dose exposure. Radiat Prot Dosimetry 104: 347–355

Raman S, Dulberg CS, Spasoff RA, and Scott T (1987) Mortality among Canadian military personnel exposed to low-dose radiation. Can Med Assoc J 136: 1051–1056

Sacher GA (1956) On the statistical nature of mortality, with especial reference to chronic radiation mortality. Radiology 67: 250–257

Sacher GA (1963) Effects of X-rays on the survival of *Drosophila* imagoes. Physiol Zool 36: 295–311

Sacher GA (1977) Life table modification and life prolongation. In: Finch CE and Hayflick L (eds) Handbook of the Biology of Aging, pp. 582–638. Van Nostrand Reinhold Co., New York

Schollnberger H, Stewart RD, Mitchel REJ and Hofmann W (2004) An examination of radiation hormesis mechanisms using a multistage carcinogenesis model. Nonlinearity Biol Toxicol Med 2: 317–352

Sheppard SC and Regitnig PJ (1987) Factors controlling the hormesis response in irradiated seed. Health Phys 52: 599–605

Shimizu Y, Pierce DA, Preston DL and Mabuchi K (1999) Studies of the mortality of atomic bomb survivors. Report 12, Part II. Noncancer mortality: 1950–1990. Radiat. Res 152: 374–389

SullivanRL and Grosch DS (1963) The radiation tolerance of an adult wasp. Nucleonics 2: 121–123

Tanaka S, Tanaka IB III, Sasagawa S, Ichinohe K, Takabatake T, Matsushita S, Matsumoto T, Otsu H and Sato F (2003) No lengthening of life span in mice continuously exposed to gamma rays at very low dose rates. Radiat Res 160: 376–379

Thompson GA, Smithers J and Boxenbaum H (1990) Biphasic mortality response of chipmunks in the wild to single doses of ionizing radiation: toxicity and longevity hormesis. Drug Metab Rev 22: 2–3

Tzschentke B and Plagemann A (2006) Imprinting and critical periods in early development. Worlds Poult Sci J 62: 626–637

Tzschentke B, Basta D and Nichelmann M (2001) Epigenetic temperature adaptation in birds: peculiarities and similarities in comparison to acclimation. News Biomed Sci 1: 26–31
UNSCEAR (1958) Report of the United Nations Scientific Committee on the Effects of Atomic Radiation. General Assembly Official Records: Thirteenth Session, Supplement No. 17 (A/3838), United Nations, New York
UNSCEAR (1994) Sources and effects of ionizing radiation, United Nations scientific committee on the effects of atomic radiation, New York
Vaiserman AM, Koshel NM, Litoshenko AY, Mozzhukhina TG and Voitenko VP (2003a) Effects of X-irradiation in early ontogenesis on the longevity and amount of the S1 nuclease-sensitive DNA sites in adult *Drosophila melanogaster*. Biogerontology 4: 9–14
Vaiserman AM, Koshel NM, Mechova LV and Voitenko VP (2004) Cross-life stage and cross-generational effects of gamma irradiations at the egg stage on *Drosophila melanogaster* life histories. Biogerontology 5: 327–337
Vaiserman AM, Litoshenko AY, Kvitnitskaia–Ryzhova TIu, Koshel NM, Mozzhukhina TG, Mikhal'skii SA and Voitenko VP (2003b) Molecular and cellular aspects of radiation hormesis in *Drosophila melanogaster*. Tsitol Genet 37: 41–48 [in Russian]
Wei LX, Zha YR, Tao ZF, He WH, Chen DQ and Yuan YL (1990) Epidemiological investigation of radiological effects in high background radiation areas of Yangjiang, China. J Radiat Res (Tokyo) 31: 119–136
Wolff S (1992) Failla memorial lecture. Is radiation all bad? The search for adaptation. Radiat Res 131: 117–123
Yeargers E (1981) Effect of gamma–radiation on dauer larvae of *Caenorhabditis elegans*. J Nematol 13: 235–237
Yoshinaga S, Mabuchi K, Sigurdson AJ, Doody MM, and Ron E (2004) Cancer risks among radiologists and radiologic technologists: review of epidemiologic studies. Radiology 233: 313–321
Zainullin VG and Moskalev AA (2001) Radiation-induced changes in the life span of laboratory Drosophila melanogaster strains. Russ J Genet 37: 1094–1095 [in Russian]
Zanchkina SI, Rozanova OM, Akhmadieva AKh, Aptikaeva GF, Klokov DIu, Smirnova EN, Zaichkin ME and Balakin VE (2002) Detection of genomic instability in offspring of male mice chronically exposed to gamma-radiation by the "adaptive response" test. Radiats Biol Radioecol 42: 608–611 [in Russian]
Zhou H, Suzuki M, Randers–Pehrson G, Vannais D, Chen G, Trosko JE, Waldren CA and Hei TK (2001) Radiation risk to low fluences of alpha particles may be greater than we thought. Proc Natl Acad Sci USA 98: 14410–14415

Chapter 4
Hypergravity in *Drosophila melanogaster*

Éric Le Bourg

Introduction

Hypergravity (HG), i.e., gravity levels higher than 1 g, the Earth gravity level, can be considered as a stress because the animal subjected to a high g-load has to adapt to a higher weight: a 3 g level means that the weight of the animal is magnified thrice. Contrarily to temperature, HG is not a natural stress, because the gravity level is constant on Earth even if one can experience slight and short HG episodes in everyday life, for instance in cars or elevators during strong braking. Therefore, while species can detect the direction of the Earth's gravity vector, for instance by using the vestibular system (see Sondag 1996), they have probably not evolved specific defense mechanisms against HG. However, even if the analogy is of a limited value, it could be said that subjecting a man weighing 70 kg to a 2 g level is like subjecting him to a 70 kg extra-weight in a backpack. This analogy is of a limited value because, in HG, the increased weight is not confined to the back but is spread on each cell of the body. Thus, even if specific defense mechanisms against HG do not exist, animals can adapt to an increased weight, as it is the case in females of mammals during pregnancy, and it can be hypothetized that they would react in HG conditions as if they were carrying an extra-weight.

Beyond the study of mild stress in flies (see below), HG has been used in mammals, mainly at the US National Aeronautics and Space Administration (NASA) during the 1960s and 1970s (Miquel and Economos 1982). In one of these studies, Economos et al. (1982) reported that rats kept at 3.14 g for life had a shorter, albeit not significant, longevity than rats kept at 1 g. Using HG in mammals is however not an easy procedure, due to technical problems. The centrifuge of the NASA, designed to study aging in rats, had a 16 m diameter (for a picture, see Oyama 1982), while that used to study the vestibular system in hamsters (for a picture, see

Centre de Recherche sur la Cognition Animale, UMR CNRS 5169, Université Paul-Sabatier, 31062 Toulouse cedex 9, France. Tel: 33 5 61 55 65 67; Fax: 33 5 61 55 61 54; e-mail: lebourg@cict.fr

E. Le Bourg and S.I.S. Rattan (eds.), *Mild Stress and Healthy Aging.*

Sondag 1996) had a 3.5 m diameter. Only a very few laboratories can use such centrifuges, due to their size. Beyond technical problems, it is worthy of note that rodents, after a severe adaptation phase during which the body weight decreases (review in Le Bourg 1999), have still some difficulty to cope with a high g-load. Hypergravity attenuates body mass gain (e.g., Kita et al. 2006) and rats exposed to 3.6 g for 21 months or to 4.7 g for 25 months show a deformation of vertebra of the thoracic cervical region with a marked lordosis (Oyama 1982). Therefore, the use of mammals to study the effect of HG on aging and longevity may face various technical and physiological issues. These physiological issues can explain why HG has not been considered in mammals as a mild stress which could have beneficial effects on aging and longevity but, rather, as a strong stress with deleterious effects. In such conditions, turning our attention to other species than mammals can be of interest.

Various mild stresses have been used in *D. melanogaster*, such as temperature (see the chapter "Temperature induced hormesis in *Drosophila*") or irradiation (see the chapter "Irradiation and hormesis"). These stresses have also been used in mammals, sometimes with conflicting results (compare Caratero et al. 1998 and Courtade et al. 2002). These mild stresses are easy to use in flies and it is possible to vary their strength. Obviously, it would be desirable to have at hand a panel of various mild stresses that can be used in the same species, allowing to compare their effects and, possibly, to draw general rules about the effects of mild stress. While non-rodent vertebrate species have sometimes been used in HG conditions (e.g., Anken et al. 1998), most of the studies using HG have been done with *D. melanogaster* in the author's laboratory and in the Genetics Laboratory of the Catholic University of Louvain-La-Neuve, Belgium. Thanks to the tiny size of *D. melanogaster*, the diameter of the centifuges used in France or in Belgium by Lints et al. (1993) was ca. 1 m. In addition, while the centrifuges designed for mammals provide only one gravity level at a time, those designed for flies allow to place vials containing animals at various distances from the axis of the centrifuge, and thus to obtain several g levels at the same time.

Studying HG in flies has other advantages. Hypergravity increases the metabolic demand of flies at the same rearing temperature, due to the higher weight. Therefore, HG is a means to increase the metabolic demand without the adverse consequences of increased temperatures in poikilotherms (increased speed of chemical reactions, decreased longevity, increased activity level, and so on). Since a fly is a holometabolous insect, its growth is complete at emergence, and thus HG cannot have any effect on its adult size, provided development occurs at 1 g (for results on development in HG, see below). Obviously, a study of the effects of HG on aging and longevity could take advantage of the other features of the fly, such as a low longevity, well-known genetics and behavioral patterns, and so on.

This article summarizes the experiments conducted in *D. melanogaster* flies subjected to HG. These results have been published between 1989 and 2005. As a first step of these studies, flies were subjected throughout life to HG. Thereafter, flies were subjected to HG only at a young age.

The First Studies: Hypergravity Throughout Lifespan Is a Strong Stress

Hypergravity is obtained by putting the usual rearing vials of flies in a continuously rotating centrifuge (Fig. 1). If the distance to the axis is increased, the HG level is also increased. With a 102 rpm speed, it is possible to obtain 1.41, 2.16, 3.02, 3.61, 3.97 and 5.02 g. Flies of the 1 g groups are on the same table as the centrifuge and are thus subjected to the same conditions as HG flies (noise, temperature, light). Two other centrifuges have been used from time to time: one, located in France, providing 1.96, 2.33, 2.72, 3.11, 3.51 and 3.92 g levels, and another one, in Belgium, providing 2.58, 3.70, 5.14, 6.31 and 7.38 g levels. Flies are subjected from the second day of imaginal life to a given g level 24 h a day (the centrifuge is briefly stopped twice a week to transfer flies to new vials containing fresh medium). In all experiments described in this chapter, except when indicated, groups of 15 virgin males or females live in 20 mL vials containing the usual medium (corn flour, agar, sugar, dead and live yeast).

Fecundity Is Modified in Hypergravity

Fecundity has been measured for life at various gravity levels in individual females kept with a single male. Since the metabolic demand is expected to increase in HG,

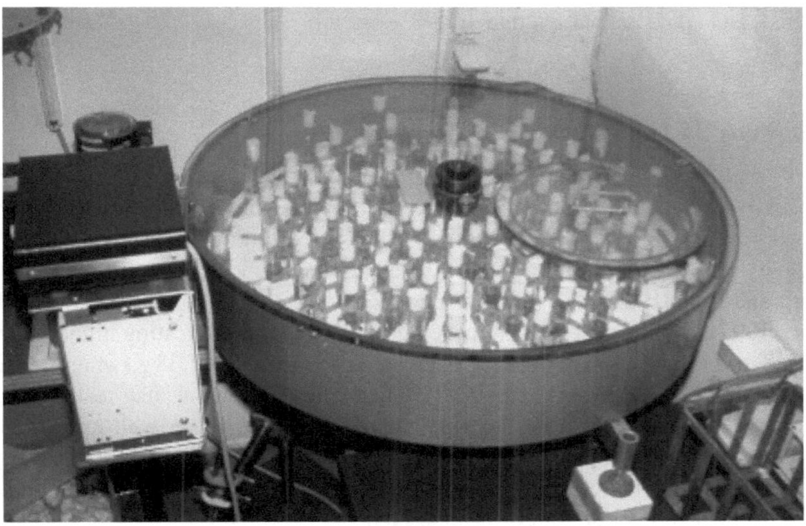

Fig. 1 Picture of the most commonly used centrifuge (1 m diameter). Flies are kept in their usual vials stored in the centrifuge. With a 102 rpm speed, the outer gravity level reaches 5 g

fecundity was expected to be modified in HG as in food restriction conditions, a rearing condition where the metabolic supply is reduced. David et al. (1971) observed that underfed females had lower lifetime, mean daily and maximal fecundities and that, with increased underfeeding, the day of maximal fecundity was delayed. Recording of individual daily fecundity in HG (1–5 g) provided similar results, except that the decrease of lifetime fecundity failed to reach significance (Lints and Le Bourg 1989). Therefore, females modulate their laying activity to cope either with a decreased metabolic supply (underfeeding) or a higher metabolic demand (HG). These first results show that living in HG is not highly detrimental to flies since they remain able to mate and lay eggs. However, the viability of their eggs could be affected by HG and it is necessary to check this point.

Viability of the Eggs Is Slightly Decreased in Hypergravity

The viability, i.e., the percentage of eggs reaching the adult stage, has been recorded to test whether HG is a stress affecting development, as it does in mammals (review in Le Bourg and Lints 1989b). Viability was recorded in eggs developing in HG (1–5 g) from parents kept at 1 g, in eggs developing at 1 g from parents kept in HG (1–5 g), and in eggs developing at the same gravity level as that used for parents (1–5 g). Hypergravity slightly decreased viability since 75% of eggs were able to reach the adult stage in the worst case (94% in the control condition: parents and eggs living at 1 g). Therefore, it can be concluded that flies can lay viable eggs in HG and that these eggs have a normal development in HG; in other words, the HG condition is not really detrimental to life. Nevertheless, even if fecundity and viability are not strongly affected, HG could decrease longevity.

Longevity Is Decreased in Hypergravity

Longevity has been recorded in several experiments. No clear deleterious effect of HG was observed in virgin flies living at a gravity level not higher than 4 g. At 5 g, longevity was shortened by around 1 week in males and 3 weeks in females (Le Bourg and Lints 1989a) but this effect could also be less important (Minois and Le Bourg 1997). Similar results were observed in an experiment testing higher g levels (1–7.38 g), both sexes having a 40 days mean longevity at 7.38 g, which is still a high value at 25 °C (Lints et al. 1993). The same experiment also tested the HG effect in mated flies. Mating strongly decreased longevity, a well-known result (Boulétreau-Merle 1988), and HG slightly decreased longevity in both sexes only above 5 g, this to a lesser extent than in virgin flies. In other words, mating by itself had a stronger impact on longevity than HG.

As for fecundity and viability, keeping flies in HG for life has some negative effect on longevity, which is however not a tragic one. It remains to know whether

HG, in addition to decrease longevity above 4 g, could also impair aging, as inferred from the study of age-related behavioral changes.

Hypergravity Seems to Accelerate Behavioral Aging

Three behaviors which are known to be affected by aging have been observed in flies of various ages living in HG (1–5 g). Flies lived in HG and were transferred at 1 g before their behavior was observed. Therefore, the behaviors were always observed at 1 g and never in HG, simply because it was impossible to observe the flies into the rotating centrifuge.

Climbing activity is the ability measured at the individual level to climb up the vertical side of a vial after having been subjected to a mechanical stimulus. The climbing score is the maximal height reached 20 s after the cessation of the mechanical stimulus. Climbing activity is impaired at older ages and this impairment was observed at younger ages in flies previously kept in HG (Le Bourg and Lints 1992a), no clear gravity effect being observed at 4 days of age.

Young flies have straight paths when they are released at the center of an arena, while older ones exhibit rather sinuous paths and do not move as far away from the center as young flies. These effects of age are increased if flies have lived in HG, no gravity effect being observed at young age (Le Bourg and Lints 1992b).

The spontaneous locomotor activity level, i.e., the number of motions recorded during a 12 h photophase, decreases with age. These effects of age are increased if flies have lived at 5 g, but no effect is observed at 3 g; no gravity effect is observed at young age (Le Bourg and Lints 1992c).

Therefore, these results show that HG seems to accelerate behavioral aging because the normal age-related changes are increased if flies have lived in HG.

However, HG does not always mimick an accelerated behavioral aging because the proboscis-extension response threshold to sucrose of males, which increases with age, is not modified if they live for 1, 4 or 7 weeks at 3 or 5 g (Le Bourg 1996). Hypergravity also decreases the speeds of habituation and learning of the inhibition of the proboscis-extension response of 1-week-old males which have lived in HG, but has no effect in middle-aged and old males that have spent 4 or 7 weeks in HG (Minois and Le Bourg 1997). These results are best explained, not by a decreased ability to learn or habituate, but rather by the consequences of an increased metabolic demand in HG inducing a mild stress to which flies must adapt. This stress was shown to have long-lasting consequences: 5 days after having been transferred at 1 g, young males still displayed a lower speed of habituation than males that always lived at 1 g (Le Bourg 1999).

In conclusion, these results on flies living permanently in HG show that HG modifies fecundity and slightly decreases viability. Longevity decreases above 4 g and behavioral aging can be accelerated in HG. It can be concluded that living in HG up to old age is rather stressful, even if not a threat to life. Since HG is a strong stress when imposed throughout life, it could be that a short stay in HG, at a young age, would act as a mild stress with possible hormetic effects. This is the rationale which prompted all the next described studies on HG.

Hypergravity at a Young Age Is a Mild Stress with Hormetic Effects

In all following experiments flies only spent a part of their life in HG, usually the first 2 weeks of adult life, but sometimes a shorter or a longer time. After the end of the stay in HG, flies were transferred to 1 g. Except when indicated, the same temperature was used into the centrifuge and at 1 g (25 °C), flies were virgin, the gravity level was in the 1–5 g range and experiments were performed in the French laboratory. The Belgian laboratory used a gravity range from 1–7.38 g.

Two Weeks in Hypergravity Increase Longevity of Males, but Not of Females

Two weeks in HG increase longevity in males (Fig. 2, +10 to 20%), but not in females, for which a negative effect of HG can exist. These results have been observed (Le Bourg and Minois 1997; Le Bourg et al. 2000, 2002) in two laboratories (France and Belgium) with two strains differing by their mean longevity at 1 g (Fig. 2b).

Since 2 weeks in HG increase longevity of males, it was of interest to vary the duration or schedule of exposure to HG. In a first experiment, flies spent a total of 12 days in HG with 4 days in HG followed by 3 days at 1 g. No positive effect of HG was observed in either sex, showing that males must be continuously exposed to HG to live longer. In the same way, a 1-week exposure to HG failed to increase longevity. By contrast, 3 weeks in HG still increased longevity in males but not 25 days, while 14, 19 and 24 days of HG exposure (1–7.38 g) increased longevity in the Belgian lab: it thus seems that 3 weeks of HG is the longer exposure which can clearly give rise to a longevity increase. This last point was checked again in a last experiment using individual rearing after transfer to 1 g, which increased longevity, particularly in males (Table 1 in Le Bourg et al. 2000). In such conditions, 25 days of HG exposure increased longevity of males (mean longevities respectively for 1, 3 and 5 g groups: 59.27, 62.60, 64.66 days). In this last experiment, while 13 days in HG increased longevity of males living in individual vials after transfer to 1 g (respectively for 1, 3 and 5 g groups: 53.78, 61.42, 61.22 days), 3 days or 46 days in HG failed to do so.

All these results (Le Bourg and Minois 1997; Le Bourg et al. 2000, 2002) show that 2 weeks in HG increase longevity of males but not of females, a shorter or intermittent exposure being inefficient. Longer exposure can also increase longevity, but this result

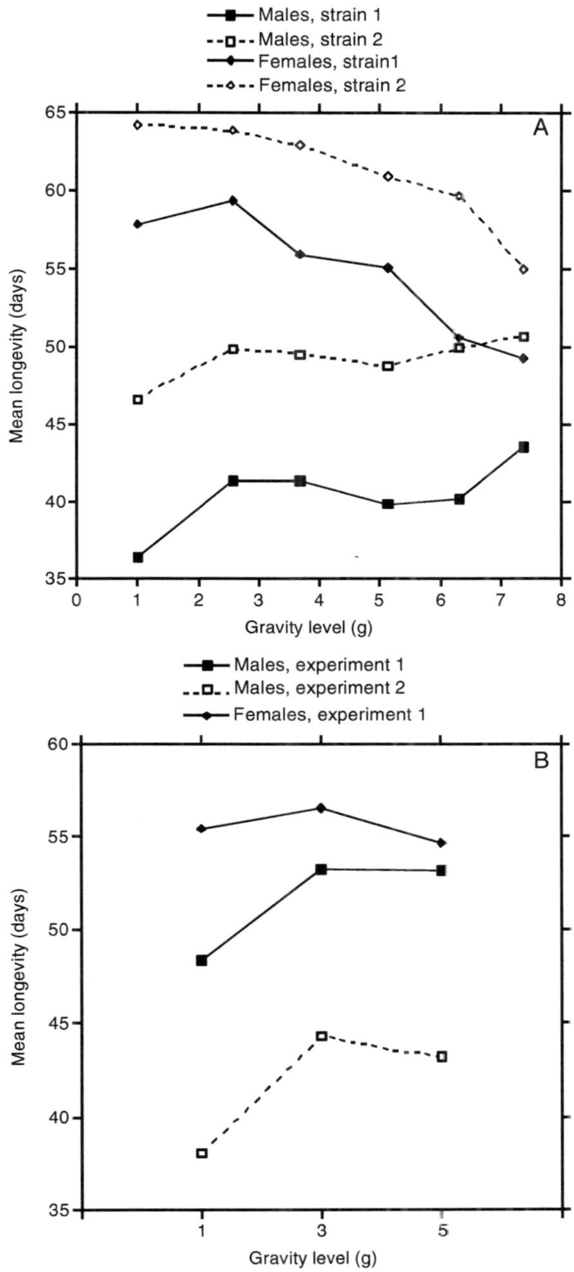

Fig. 2 Effect of a 2-week stay in HG, from the second day of adult life, on longevity of *D. melanogaster.* A. Two wild-type strains, differing by their mean longevity at 1 g, are used in a Belgian laboratory (Le Bourg et al. 2000). Each point is the mean of ca. 145 flies. B. The strain 2 (wild-type strain Meyzieu) is tested with another centrifuge in a French laboratory. The figure reports two experiments for which the longevity at 1 g was contrasted (Le Bourg et al. 2000, 2002). Each point is the mean of ca. 60 (experiment 1) or 100 flies (experiment 2)

is not stable, as it depends on the rearing condition (individual vs group rearing) and on experiments. It seems probable that 3 weeks in HG are the limit between a mild stress with hormetic effect and a strong stress with no such effect (see the chapter "What is hormesis?" for a discussion of the hormetic dose–response relationship).

As a matter of fact, the positive effect of HG on longevity can disappear if flies are subjected to a too strong stress. Mating is known to decrease longevity (Boulétreau-Merle 1988): in mated males, 2 weeks in HG have no positive effect on longevity, which indicates that subjecting flies to a living condition decreasing longevity can suppress the positive effect of HG. Similar conclusions can be reached if flies are transferred after a 2-week stay in HG at 28 °C or 30 °C: no positive HG effect on longevity of males is observed in these conditions shortening longevity (Le Bourg et al. 2004). This result is exactly the contrary of what was expected by Sacher (1977), who wrote that hormetic effects are "unlikely to occur in the healthy active individual, and are more likely to be significant in the ill or depressed animal".

These results on longevity thus show that HG may have a hormetic effect on longevity. It is of interest to know whether similar effects are observed on behavioral aging.

Two Weeks in Hypergravity May Delay Behavioral Aging, Mainly in Males

The same behaviors as those previously observed during the study of HG throughout life (see above) have been used.

Flies kept in HG for 2 weeks displayed a lower climbing score than those always kept at 1 g the day following transfer to 1 g, but higher scores some days after this transfer (Fig. 3, Le Bourg and Minois 1999; Le Bourg et al. 2002), all flies being unable to climb up the side of the vial at 5 weeks of age. This effect is mainly observed in males, but a positive effect of HG may also be shown in females. No positive effect of HG has been observed if flies were kept in HG for only the first week of adult life or for 4 weeks (Minois 1998). However, it is difficult to conclude anything from this last experiment, because climbing scores are very low in flies older than 4 weeks of age.

Old flies released at the center of a circular arena exhibit rather sinuous paths and do not move as far away as young flies. At old age, flies kept in HG for 2 weeks at young age moved more away the center of the arena than flies always kept at 1 g, but HG had no effect on the sinuosity of the path (Le Bourg and Minois 1999). There is thus only a slight tendency for a slower behavioral aging if flies have lived in HG at a young age.

By contrast, having lived in HG for 2 weeks at young age had no positive effect on spontaneous locomotor activity level at old age, i.e., the number of motions recorded during a 12 h photophase (Le Bourg and Minois 1999).

All these results indicate that, depending on the studied behavior, a 2-week stay in HG at young age can delay behavioral aging or has no effect on it. Thus, HG can increase longevity of males and delay aging: could it also protect against strong stresses?

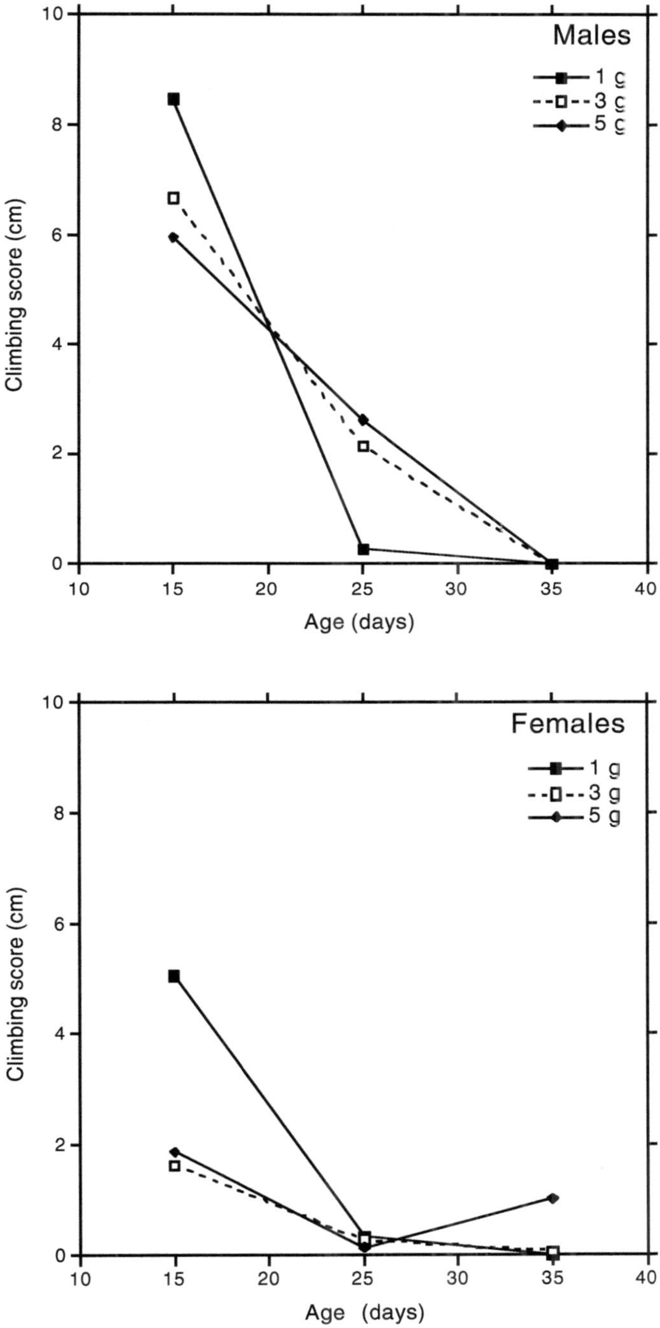

Fig. 3 Effect of a 2-week stay in HG, from the second day of adult life, on climbing scores of *D. melanogaster*, i.e., the ability, measured at the individual level, to climb up the vertical side of a vial after having been subjected to a mechanical stimulus (Le Bourg et al. 2002). The climbing score is the maximal height reached in 20 s after the cessation of the mechanical stimulus. Each point is the mean of 15 flies

One to 4 Weeks in Hypergravity Increase Survival Time to Heat but have no Effect on Other Stresses

A mild stress may increase resistance to a strong stress. For instance, a mild heat or cold stress increases survival time to heat (see the chapter "Temperature induced hormesis in *Drosophila*"). Similarly, spending 2 weeks in HG at a young age increases survival time at 37 °C in both sexes (Fig. 4). Other experiments, using either 1, 2 or 4 weeks of HG exposure starting the second day of life provided similar results, but no HG effect was observed with a 7 weeks exposure (Le Bourg and Minois 1997; Le Bourg et al. 2002; Minois and Le Bourg 1999; Minois et al. 1999).

Could this effect of HG on heat resistance be explained by a behavioral adaptation to heat? Indeed, flies previously kept in HG could be more inactive at 37 °C than flies always kept at 1 g: this reduced locomotor activity, a costly metabolic activity, could explain their higher survival time. Spontaneous locomotor activity was individually recorded at 37 °C until death in flies which spent 1 week in HG (Minois and Le Bourg 1999). These flies survived longer at 37 °C than those always kept at 1 g but the mean activity level did not vary with the gravity level (1, 3, 5 g), which shows that the high survival of flies which have lived in HG is not explained

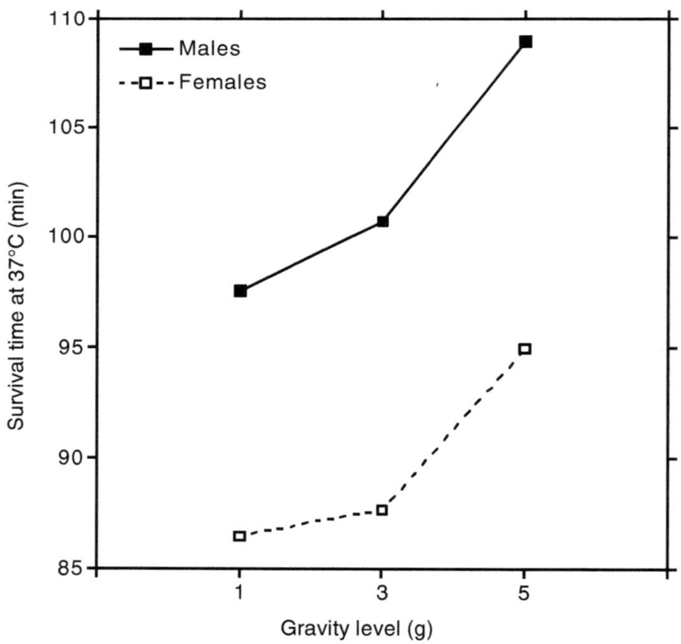

Fig. 4 Effect of a 2-week stay in HG, from the second day of adult life, on survival time at 37 °C of *D. melanogaster*. Flies are placed in tight vials in a waterbath set at 37 °C and the number of dead flies is recorded every 5 min up to the death of the last fly. Each point is the mean of ca. 45 flies

by a decreased energy expenditure. Furthermore, in each sex and gravity group, the individual activity score was positively correlated with survival time. In other words, in each sex and gravity group, flies which survived longer were also more active.

The positive effect of HG on heat resistance cannot be extended to other stresses because HG has no effect on resistance to cold (0 °C), desiccation and starvation (Minois and Le Bourg 1999).

Two Weeks in Hypergravity Help Middle-Aged Males to Cope with Simulated Heatwave

Flies kept in HG at a young age survive longer at 37 °C than flies always kept at 1 g (Fig. 4). While this result is of interest, it would be still more interesting if HG could also help to recover from a deleterious but non lethal heat stress, such as a sudden but transient temperature rise. These transient temperature rises have been of a tragic importance for elderly people during the 2003 summer heatwave.

To simulate heatwave, flies have been subjected to a 37 °C stress for 60 or 90 min, a duration decreasing longevity (–50%) after the heat shock, but not killing flies, since most of them survived to these rather long heat shocks. Males heat-shocked at 4 weeks of age which lived 2 weeks in HG at a young age survived 15% longer than 1 g ones (Fig. 5). No positive effect of HG was observed at 5 or 6 weeks of age and in 4- to 6-week-old females. The heat shock decreased climbing activity and spontaneous locomotor activity scores but HG did not counteract this effect at any age and in any sex. Therefore, HG protects against a deleterious non lethal heat shock but not against the behavioral impairments due to this shock (Le Bourg et al. 2004).

This experiment was reiterated using several shocks of a shorter duration. Flies were subjected from 4 weeks of age to 4 heat shocks (30 or 45 min at 37 °C) during a 2-week period. Males that spent 2 weeks in HG at a young age lived 15% longer than flies always kept at 1 g, no effect being observed in females (Fig. 6). Furthermore, living in HG had nearly no effect on the longevity difference between the HG and the 1 g groups when the deleterious effect of heat was moderate, i.e., when the longevity of 1 g groups was not strongly shortened by heat. By contrast, males took advantage of a stay in HG if the negative effect of heat was important (Le Bourg 2005). Therefore, these results show that a mild stress applied at young age protects against a strong stress at middle age.

In conclusion, this whole set of results shows that HG at a young age has hormetic effects on longevity, provided HG exposure is not too short or long and the rearing conditions do not decrease longevity. Hormetic effects are also observed on behavioral aging (but not on all studied behavioral traits), and on resistance to heat (but not to other stresses). Hypergravity can thus help flies, particularly males, to live a better old age and it is now of concern to know the possible mechanisms of these effects.

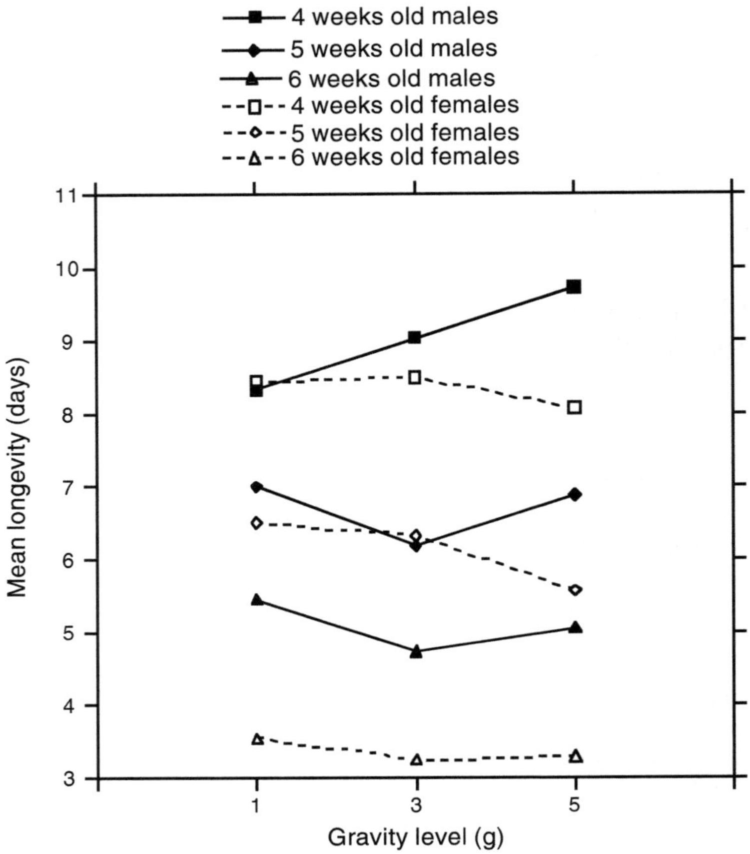

Fig. 5 Effect of a 2-week stay in HG, from the second day of adult life, on longevity of *D. melanogaster* after a 60 or 90 min 37 °C heat shock. Day 0 is the day of shock and the 60 and 90 min groups are pooled in the figure. Flies were either 4-, 5- or 6-week old the day of heat shock. Each point is the mean, respectively at 4, 5 and 6 weeks of age, of 133–170, 107–165, and 94–147 flies

A Search for the Mechanisms of the Hormetic Effects of Hypergravity

A mild stress, i.e., a low dose of an otherwise deleterious stimulus is expected to upregulate maintenance and repair pathways to induce hormesis (see the chapter "What is hormesis?"). Studies on two kinds of such repair pathways have been done in flies subjected to HG: the antioxidant enzymes superoxide dismutase (SOD) and catalase (CAT), on the one hand, and the 70 kDa heat shock protein on the other hand.

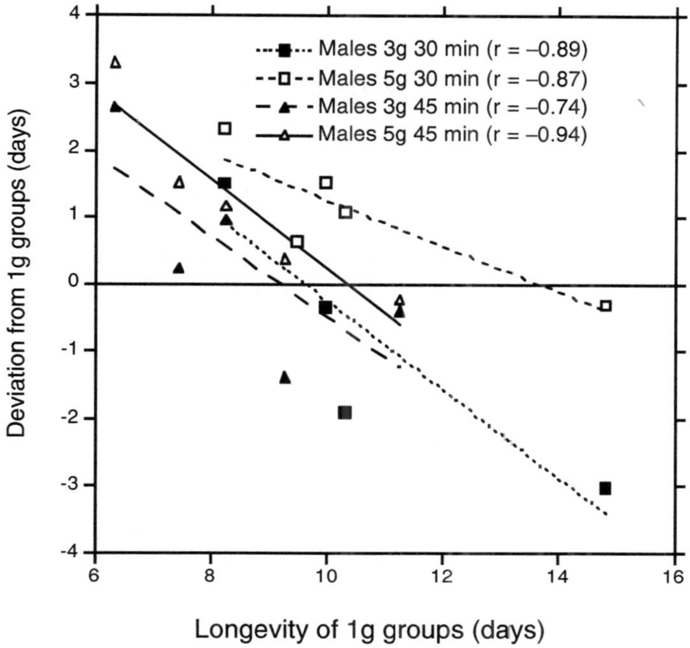

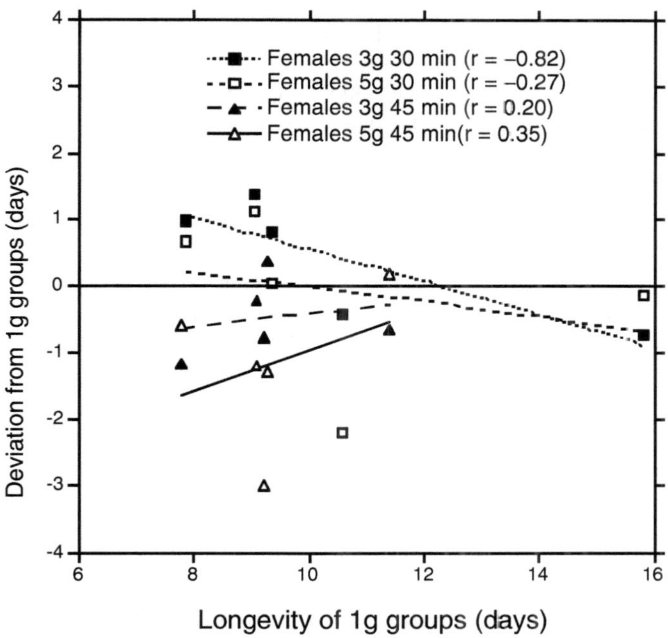

Fig. 6 Effect of a 2-week stay in HG, from the second day of adult life, on longevity of *D. melanogaster* after 4 heat shocks (30 or 45 min at 37 °C) during a 2-week period starting at 4 weeks of age. The figure shows the difference between the mean longevity of flies which lived at 3 or 5 g and that of flies always living at 1 g. For each length of heat shock, five replicates were done (total n = 2,352). Each point stands for the mean of a replicate

Antioxidant Enzymes Do Not Explain the Hormetic Effects of Hypergravity

According to the well-known free radical theory of aging (Harman 1956), aging is explained by the damages due to the free radicals produced during normal metabolism, despite the existence of antioxidant defenses. If this theory is correct, one may expect that a higher activity of antioxidant enzymes, for instance in transgenic flies overexpressing SOD or CAT, could increase longevity (review in, e.g., Sohal et al. 2002).

Since flies weigh more in HG than at 1 g, their metabolic rate could be increased in HG: the egg-laying activity decreases in flies living in HG as in food-restricted flies (see above), which suggests that the metabolic demand increases in HG. The metabolic rate of flies has not been measured in HG but a higher metabolism has been reported in HG-adapted rats than in 1 g ones (Oyama and Chan 1973; Daligcon and Oyama 1975; Wade et al. 2002). One could thus hypothetize that a higher metabolic rate of flies in HG could induce a higher activity of antioxidant enzymes in order to counteract an increased production of free radicals during the oxidative phosphorylation process. As an outcome, flies that have lived in HG could be more protected against free radical attacks than those always living at 1 g and, if this protection would persist after removal from HG, they could better resist free radicals and live longer. However, a longer life would be observed only if antioxidant defenses do have a beneficial effect on longevity, as postulated by the free radical theory (Harman 1956).

The first step to test this hypothesis is to measure the activity of antioxidant enzymes in flies that have lived in HG. SOD and CAT were measured in homogenates of individual males and females that have lived at various gravity levels (1, 3, 5 g) for the first 2 weeks of adult life. The enzymatic activity was measured at 2, 4, or 6 weeks of age, i.e., just after transfer from HG to 1 g, and 2 or 4 weeks later: the gravity level had no effect on SOD and CAT at any age and in any sex (Le Bourg and Fournier 2004).

Therefore, flies that have lived in HG are not better protected against free radical attacks than flies always living at 1 g. This result is in accordance with that of Niedzwiecki et al. (1992) who showed that a 37 °C heat shock had no clear effect on SOD and CAT activities in 2-, 24-, or 50-day-old male flies. Even if other antioxidant defenses, such as reduced glutathione, have not been measured in our studies it seems that the increased longevity of males is not linked to an increased activity of antioxidant enzymes. Since antioxidant enzymes appear not to explain the hormetic effects of HG, it is therefore needed to focus on another repair pathway, the heat shock proteins.

The 70 kDa Heat Shock Protein Could Explain the Hypergravity Effect on Heat Resistance but Not That on Longevity

Heat shock proteins (Hsp) are molecular chaperones, differing by their molecular weight, which are induced by various stresses in *D. melanogaster* and other species (review in Morrow and Tanguay 2003). In *D. melanogaster*, the 70 kDa Hsp (Hsp70) is expressed, for instance, after a heat (e.g., Dahlgaard et al. 1998) or cold shock (Sejerkilde et al. 2003, but see also Overgaard et al. 2005). It is known that heat or cold shocks can increase longevity and resistance to some stresses, particularly in *D. melanogaster* (see the chapter "Temperature induced hormesis in *Drosophila*"). Therefore, Hsp70 could explain the hormetic effects of temperature stresses on longevity. Could a higher expression of Hsp70 also explain the hormetic effects of HG on longevity, resistance to heat and behavioral aging?

A first study (Western immunoblot procedure) measured Hsp70 expresssion in flies that lived in HG (3 or 5 g) for 1, 4 or 7 weeks before to be transferred at 1 g (Minois et al. 1999). An antibody against both the inducible and constitutive (i.e., expressed even in the absence of heat shock) forms of Hsp70 was available for this study. The comparison of the size of the blots showed that, in each sex, HG did not increase Hsp70 expresssion at any age. By contrast, flies kept in HG for 2 weeks from the second day of adult life and subjected to a heat shock (60 min at 37 °C) after their transfer at 1 g had a higher synthesis of Hsp70. Thus, HG by itself did not provoke Hsp70 synthesis, even after 7 weeks in HG, but more Hsp70 was expressed after a heat shock if flies were kept in HG before this heat shock. This study has been replicated using an antibody against the inducible form of Hsp70 only. It was confirmed (Fig. 7) that HG does not provoke Hsp70 synthesis but that more protein is synthetized after a heat shock (45 min at 37 °C) if flies lived for 2 weeks in HG at young age (Le Bourg et al. 2002).

The HG-linked increased heat resistance could thus be explained by an increased Hsp70 synthesis. However, the increased longevity or delayed behavioral aging of flies that lived in HG for 2 weeks cannot be explained by Hsp70 because this protein is not synthetized at 25 °C, the rearing temperature of flies, even after 1, 2, 4 or 7 weeks in HG. Since Hsp70 probably explains a part of the HG effects, one may wonder whether transgenic flies overexpressing *hsp70* would take advantage of more Hsp70 synthesis when subjected to HG.

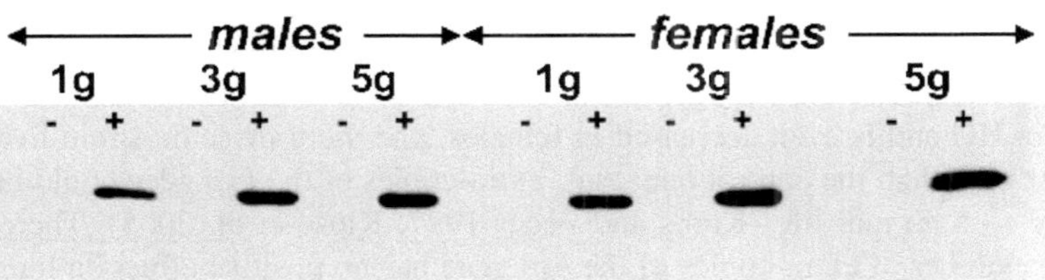

Fig. 7 Effect of a 2-week stay in HG, from the second day of adult life, on Hsp70 expression of *D. melanogaster* after a heat shock (45 min at 37 °C: + on the figure) or no heat shock (– on the figure). Fifteen flies were used for each blot

Overexpression of the 70 kDa Heat Shock Protein does not Increase the Hypergravity Effect on Heat Resistance and has no Effect on Longevity or Behavioral Aging

Thanks to transgenesis technics, flies overexpressing *hsp70* are available (Welte et al. 1993). Since HG increases Hsp70 synthesis when flies are subjected to a heat shock, it could be hypothetized that these transgenic flies would take more advantage of a stay in HG than control ones.

The longevity of flies which have lived for 1 or 2 weeks in HG (3 or 5 g) at young age was recorded in a transgenic strain with 12 extra-copies of the *hsp70* gene or in a control strain harboring the transfection vector but no extra-copies (Le Bourg et al. 2002). In both strains, no positive effect of HG was observed in males and HG decreased longevity of females. The experiment was reiterated with males only, flies being transferred to individual vials after 1 or 2 weeks in HG, which increased longevity (+50%). Here again, no positive effect of HG on longevity was observed in either strain. In all experiments, the transgenic strain lived for a shorter time than the control one. A control experiment, carried out at the same time as the experiments with the transgenic and control strains, showed that males of the wild strain used in most of experiments described in this article lived longer if they spent 2 weeks in HG. Thus, the absence of a positive HG effect on longevity in the transgenic and control strains is really strain-specific. It could be that the transgenic and control strains suffer from a heavy genetic load obscuring the positive effects of HG on longevity observed in wild-type strains (Fig. 2), because the transgenic and control strains are derived from an inbred strain. In accordance with this hypothesis, no positive effect of HG on climbing activity at middle age was observed in these strains, while such an effect was observed in the usual wild strain (Fig. 3).

By contrast, 1 or 2 weeks in HG increased survival time at 37 °C in both transgenic and control strains. This effect was due to males only (Fig. 8). Furthermore, the transgenic strain survived longer at 37 °C than the control strain at 1 week of age, but no strain effect was observed at 2 weeks of age. The positive effect of the extra-copies of the *hsp* gene on survival to heat is thus transient. Finally, HG increased survival time at 37 °C to the same extent in males of both transgenic and control strains (Fig. 8), showing that extra-copies of the *hsp70* gene increase survival time at 37 °C, but not the positive effect of HG on survival time.

This whole set of results shows that the positive effects of HG on survival time at 37 °C are not increased in flies carrying extra-copies of the *hsp* gene. The longevity of the males of the transgenic and control strains is not increased after having lived in HG and is even decreased in females, and the transgenic strain lives for a shorter time than the control one: thus, extra-copies of the *hsp* gene could be detrimental to a normal life (Krebs and Feder 1997; Klose et al. 2005). Therefore, a higher number of extra-copies of the *hsp* gene has no positive effect on longevity.

Furthermore, HG increases survival time at 37 °C and has no positive effect on longevity of these transgenic and control strains. This result observed in females of the usual wild strain (compare Figs. 2 and 4) is thus also shown in both sexes of the transgenic and control strains. The effects of HG on survival to heat and longevity

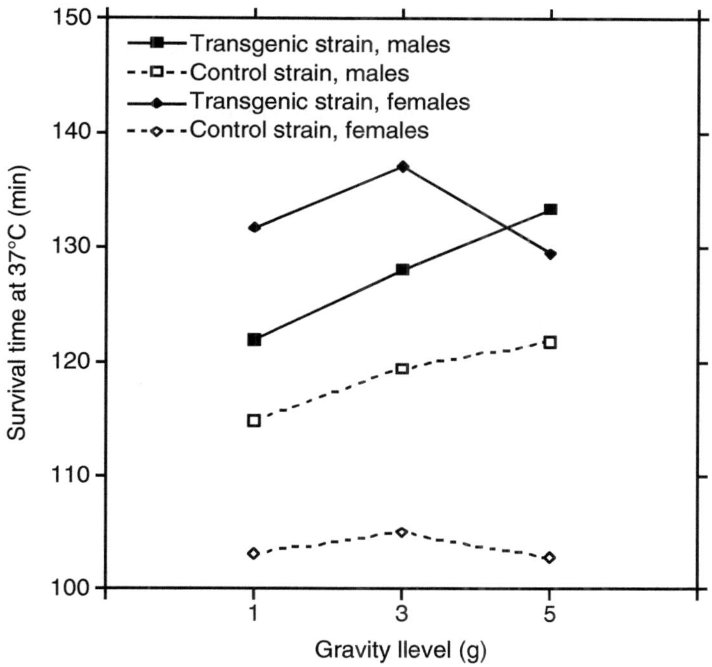

Fig. 8 Effect of a 1-week stay in HG, from the second day of adult life, on survival time at 37 °C of *D. melanogaster* transgenic and control strains. The transgenic strain has 12 extra-copies of the *hsp70* gene. Flies are placed in tight vials in a waterbath set at 37 °C and the number of dead flies is recorded every 5 min up to the death of the last fly. Each point is the mean of ca. 45 flies

are thus probably not due to a single cause: the increased resistance to heat is probably linked to the increased synthesis of Hsp70, while the cause of the increased longevity remains unknown.

In conclusion, these studies have shown that the HG effects on longevity, behavioral aging and resistance to heat are not explained by an increased activity of the antioxidant enzymes SOD and CAT. The increased synthesis of Hsp70 can probably explain, at least partly, the increased resistance to heat but not the effects on longevity and behavioral aging, since Hsp70 is not synthetized at 25 °C. Therefore, the cause of the HG effects on these traits remains unknown and more research on this question is needed.

General Conclusion: Hypergravity As a Mild Stress with Hormetic Effects on Aging, Longevity and Heat Resistance

Spending 2 weeks in HG at a young age has beneficial effects on longevity (in males), behavioral aging (mainly in males) and survival time at 37 °C (in both sexes). Furthermore, males subjected to HG at young age live longer after non-lethal heat shocks occurring at middle age. The cause of the two first effects remains unknown while the increased resistance to heat seems to be linked to an increased Hsp70 synthesis.

Hypergravity is thus a good example of a mild stress with hormetic effects on aging and longevity but, as emphasized in the introduction of this article, it probably cannot be used to study hormesis and aging in mammals. However, this study of HG shows the possible effects of a mild stress in an organism. Other studies of mild stress in *D. melanogaster* carried out in the same laboratory and with the same strain have shown that mild heat shocks at young age could also, but very slightly, increase longevity. This study also reported a longer survival at 37 °C after mild heat shocks, but not a delayed behavioral aging (Le Bourg et al. 2001). Cold shocks at young age also increase longevity and survival time at 37 °C, decrease the deleterious effects of non-lethal heat or cold shocks on longevity, and delay an age-related behavioral change (Le Bourg 2007a). Finally, if middle-aged flies feed on a sucrose solution, a poorly nutritious medium which strongly decreases longevity, a low dose of hydrogen peroxide added to this solution reduces its negative effect on longevity (Le Bourg 2007b). This result shows that a low dose of a harmful chemical can be beneficial in some conditions.

Therefore, various mild stresses have positive effects on aging, longevity, and resistance to stress in *D. melanogaster*, but these effects are dependent on the mild stress used to provoke hormesis. For the time being, *D. melanogaster* is the species for which there is the most extended database on the effects of mild stress on aging. Since various mild stresses have rather similar positive effects on aging, it seems inescapable to conclude that hormetic effects on aging do exist and that they can be observed easily, provided the experimenter is able to identify the mild stress to use. One can thus hypothetize that hormesis has been selected during the course of evolution as a means to protect against strong stresses occurring at young age but, since in the wild most of animals do not live up to old age, it was not used to protect the old organism or to increase its longevity. Thanks to laboratory rearing methods allowing flies to live up to old age, it is possible to show that hormetic effects can also be observed at old age. Hormesis thus appears to be a rescue system designed to be used at young age that can be also used at old age, even if, in the wild, it is never used at this age due to the death at an early age of most of animals.

The antagonistic pleiotropy theory of aging (Williams 1957, review in Le Bourg 2001) tells us that alleles may have beneficial effects at young age and deleterious ones at old age, and that these undesired effects have not been selected against. There is no selection against these deleterious effects simply because at old age a very few animals are still alive and reproduce and, thus, alleles provoking such effects cannot be eliminated from the gene pool. The hormesis results seem to indicate that a rescue system used at young age can be used at old age, i.e., that favorable effects at old age have not been selected for. These favorable effects at old age have not been selected because only very few animals are still alive at this age. In a way, there is thus some irony regarding side-effects occurring at old age of the natural selection process: provided an animal is able to reach old age, side-effects of genes selected for their effects at young age may reveal to be favorable (hormesis) or not (antagonistic pleiotropy).

If the existence of hormesis can be linked to a selection process of a rescue system used at young age by various species (Minois 2000), hormetic effects at old age are probably not present only in a single species, *D. melanogaster*. Since various mild stresses have rather similar positive effects in the fly, one may wonder whether there is some hope to extend the conclusion that mild stress is beneficial to aging, longevity and resistance to strong stresses not only to other poikilotherms (e.g., in the nematode, Cypser and Johnson 2002), but also to mammals. The panel of effects observed in *D. melanogaster* is rather large, which warrants to search for stresses having similar effects in mammals. While exercise has beneficial effects on aging and longevity of mammals, including human beings (see the chapter "Physical activity: a strong stimulant for hormesis during aging"), it is necessary to discover other mild stresses than exercise because it would be of interest to have at hand several mild stresses with hormetic effects in mammals. As emphasized in the introduction of this chapter, HG cannot be such a stress for mammals, and particularly human beings, for technical and physiological reasons. However, it can be expected that, since HG, temperature (chapter "Temperature induced hormesis in *Drosophila*"), and irradiation (chapter "Irradiation and hormesis") have beneficial effects on the aging of *D. melanogaster*, several stresses could be efficient in mammals, too. Obviously, if hormesis would remain confined to lower species, it would be a very interesting phenomenon but of no application to prevent age-related diseases and maintain physical and mental abilities. The issues to resolve to use hormesis in therapy are thus important (Rattan 2004) and only experimental work will tell us whether using mild stress in aging research was a good idea or not.

References

Anken RH, Ibsch M, Rahmann H (1998) Neurobiology of fish under altered gravity conditions. Brain Res Rev 28:9–18

Boulétreau-Merle J (1988) Biological factors. In Lints FA, Soliman MH (eds) Drosophila as a model organism for ageing studies. Blackie, Glasgow, pp.85–96

Caratero A, Courtade M, Bonnet L, Planel H, Caratero C (1998) Effect of a continuous gamma irradiation at a very low dose on the life span of mice. Gerontology 44:272–276

Courtade M, Billotet C, Gasset G, Caratero A, Charlet JP, Pipy B, Caratero C (2002) Life span, cancer and non-cancer diseases in mouse exposed to a continuous very low dose of gamma-irradiation. Intl J Radiat Biol 78:845–855

Cypser JR, Johnson TE (2002) Multiple stressors in Caenorhabditis elegans induce stress hormesis and extended longevity. J Gerontol Biol Sci 57A:B109–B114

Dahlgaard J, Loeschcke V, Michalak P, Justesen J (1998) Induced thermotolerance and associated expression of the heat-shock protein Hsp70 in adult Drosophila melanogaster. Funct Ecol 12:786–793

Daligcon BC, Oyama J (1975) Increased uptake and utilization of glucose by diaphragms of rats exposed to chronic centrifugation. Am J Physiol 228:742–746

David J, Van Herrewege J, Fouillet P (1971) Quantitative under-feeding of Drosophila: Effects on adult longevity and fecundity. Exp Geront 6:249–257

Economos AC, Miquel J, Ballard RC, Blemden M, Lindseth KA, Fleming J, Philpott DE, Oyama J (1982) Effects of simulated increased gravity on the rate of aging of rats. Implications for the rate of living theory of aging. Arch Gerontol Geriatr 1:349–363

Harman D (1956) Aging: A theory based on free radical and radiation chemistry. J Geront 11:298–300

Kita S, Shibata S, Kim H, Otsubo A, Ito M, Iwasaki KI (2006) Dose-dependent effects of hypergravity on body mass in mature rats. Aviat Space Environ Med 77:842–845

Klose MK, Chu D, Xiao C, Seroude L, Robertson RM (2005) Heat-shock-mediated thermoprotection of larval locomotion compromised by ubiquitous overexpression of Hsp70 in Drosophila melanogaster. J Neurophysiol 94:3563–3572

Krebs RA, Feder ME (1997) Deleterious consequences of Hsp70 overexpression in Drosophila melanogaster larvae. Cell Stress Chap 2:60–71

Le Bourg E (1996) Hypergravity and aging in *Drosophila melanogaster*. 8. Proboscis-extension-response threshold to sucrose. Gerontology 42:235–240

Le Bourg E (1999) A review of the effects of microgravity and of hypergravity on aging and longevity. Exp Geront 34:319–336

Le Bourg E (2001) A mini-review of the evolutionary theories of aging. Is it the time to accept them? Demogr Res 4:1–28

Le Bourg E (2005) Hormetic protection of Drosophila melanogaster middle-aged male flies from heat stress by mildly stressing them at young age. Naturwiss 92:293–296

Le Bourg E (2007a) Positive effects of exposure to cold at young age on longevity, aging and reistance to heat or cold shocks in Drosophila melanogaster. Biogerontology 8: 431–444

Le Bourg E (2007b) Hormetic effects on longevity of hydrogen peroxide in Drosophila melanogaster flies living on a poorly nutritious medium. Biogerontology 8: 327–344

Le Bourg E, Fournier D (2004) Is lifespan extension accompanied by improved antioxidant defences? A study of superoxide dismutase and catalase in *Drosophila melanogaster* flies that lived in hypergravity at young age. Biogeront 5:261–266

Le Bourg E, Lints FA (1989a) Hypergravity and ageing in *Drosophila melanogaster*. 2. Longevity. Gerontology 35:244–252

Le Bourg E, Lints FA (1989b) Hypergravity and ageing in *Drosophila melanogaster*. 3. Viability. Gerontology 35:253–259

Le Bourg E, Lints FA (1992a) Hypergravity and ageing in *Drosophila melanogaster*. 4. Climbing activity. Gerontology 38:59–64

Le Bourg E, Lints FA (1992b) Hypergravity and ageing in *Drosophila melanogaster*. 5. Patterns of movement. Gerontology 38:65–70

Le Bourg E, Lints FA (1992c) Hypergravity and ageing in *Drosophila melanogaster*. 6. Spontaneous locomotor activity. Gerontology 38:71–79

Le Bourg E, Minois N (1997) Increased longevity and resistance to heat shock in *Drosophila melanogaster* flies exposed to hypergravity. C R Acad Sci Paris 320:215–221

Le Bourg E, Minois N (1999) A mild stress, hypergravity exposure, postpones behavioral aging in *Drosophila melanogaster*. Exp Geront 34:157–172

Le Bourg E, Minois N, Bullens P, Baret P (2000) A mild stress due to hypergravity exposure at young age increases longevity in *Drosophila melanogaster* males. Biogeront 1:145–155

Le Bourg E, Toffin E, Massé A (2004) Male *Drosophila melanogaster* flies exposed to hypergravity at young age are protected against a non-lethal heat shock at middle age but not against behavioral impairments due to this shock. Biogeront 5:431–443

Le Bourg E,Valenti P, Lucchetta P, Payre F (2001) Effects of mild heat shocks at young age on aging and longevity in *Drosophila melanogaster*. Biogeront 2:155–164

Le Bourg E, Valenti P, Payre F (2002) Lack of hypergravity-associated longevity extension in *Drosophila melanogaster* flies overexpressing hsp70. Biogeront 3:355–364

Lints FA, Bullens P, Le Bourg E (1993) Hypergravity and aging in Drosophila melanogaster. 7. New longevity data. Exp Geront 28:611–615

Lints FA, Le Bourg E (1989) Hypergravity and ageing in *Drosophila melanogaster*. 1. Fecundity. Gerontology 35:235–243

Minois N (1998) Stress modéré et vieilllissement chez Drosophila melanogaster: mise en évidence d'effets bénéfiques d'une exposition à l'hypergravité. Doctoral dissertation, University Paul-Sabatier, Toulouse

Minois N (2000) Longevity and aging: Beneficial effects of exposure to mild stress. Biogeront 1:15–29

Minois N, Le Bourg E (1997) Hypergravity and aging in Drosophila melanogaster. 9. Conditioned suppression and habituation of the proboscis extension response. Aging Clin Exp Res 9:281–291

Minois N, Le Bourg E (1999) Resistance to stress as a function of age in *Drosophila melanogaster* living in hypergravity. Mech Ageing Dev 109:53–64

Minois N, Guinaudy MJ, Payre F, Le Bourg E (1999) HSP70 induction may explain the long-lasting resistance to heat of *Drosophila melanogaster* having lived in hypergravity. Mech Ageing Dev 109:65–77

Miquel J, Economos AC (1982) Space gerontology (eds.). Nasa Conference Publication 2248

Morrow G, Tanguay RM (2003) Heat shock proteins and aging in Drosophila melanogaster. Seminars Cell Develop Biol 14:291–299

Niedzwiecki A, Reveillaud I, Fleming JE (1992) Changes in superoxide dismutase and catalase in heat-shocked Drosophila. Free Rad Res Comms 17:355–367

Overgaard J, Sorensen JG, Petersen SO, Loeschcke V, Holmstrup M (2005) Changes in membrane lipid following rapid cold hardening in Drosophila melanogaster. J Insect Physiol 51:1173–1182

Oyama J (1982) Metabolic effects of hypergravity on experimental animals. In Miquel J, Economos AC (eds.) Space gerontology. Nasa Conference Publication 2248, pp. 37–51

Oyama J, Chan L (1973) Oxygen consumption and carbon dioxide production in rats during acute centrifugation stress and after adaptation to chronic centrifugation. Fed Proc 32:392–392

Rattan SIS (2004) Aging intervention, prevention, and therapy through hormesis. J Geront Biol Sci 59A:705–709

Sacher GA (1977) Life table modification and life prolongation. In Finch CE, Hayflick L (eds.) Handbook of the biology of aging. Van Nostrand Reinhold Co., New York

Sejerkilde M, Sorensen JG, Loeschcke V (2003) Effects of cold- and heat hardening on thermal resistance in Drosophila melanogaster. J Insect Physiol 49:719–726

Sohal RS, Mockett RJ, Orr WC (2002) Mechanisms of aging: An appraisal of the oxidative stress hypothesis. Free Rad Biol Med 33:575–586

Sondag E (1996) The effects of hypergravity on function and structure of the peripheral vestibular system. Ph.D. thesis, University of Amsterdam

Wade CE, Moran MM, Oyama J (2002) Resting energy expenditure of rats acclimated to hypergravity. Aviat Space Environ Med 73:859–864

Welte MA, Tetrault JM, Dellavalle RP, Lindquist SL (1993) A new method for manipulating transgenes: Engineering heat tolerance in a complex, multicellular organism. Curr Biol 3:842–853

Williams GC (1957) Pleiotropy, natural selection and the evolution of senescence. Evolution 11:398–411

Chapter 5
Temperature-Induced Hormesis in *Drosophila*

Jesper G. Sørensen[1], Pernille Sarup[1], Torsten N. Kristensen[1,2] and Volker Loeschcke[1]

Introduction

The phenomenon that a mild exposure to an otherwise detrimental stress factor can be beneficial, termed hormesis, is well known for many organisms and life-history traits (Khazaeli et al. 1997; Le Bourg and Minois 1997; Bubliy et al. 1998; Minois 2000; Parsons 2000). Mild stress treatments have been shown to induce hormesis in mammals and insects (Rattan 1998; Minois 2000; Le Bourg et al. 2001; Hercus et al. 2003) and increased performance has been reported with respect to, e.g., delayed aging, increased longevity and (heat) resistance to severe stress long after the hormesis inducing stress was applied (Le Bourg and Minois 1999; Hercus et al. 2003, as exemplified in Fig. 1). Thus, mild stress exposure may have long-lasting effects, much longer than the vast majority of the stress-induced changes in metabolites, proteins and gene expression (Dahlgaard et al. 1998; Sørensen et al. 2005; Malmendal et al. 2006).

High temperature is one of the stress factors that has been shown to induce hormesis (Rattan 1998; Le Bourg et al. 2001; Hercus et al. 2003; Kristensen et al. 2003; Scannapieco et al. 2007). The reason for choosing high temperature as a model stress is that it is easy to expose experimental organisms to well-defined thermal regimes and because it is a natural occurring stress for many plant and animal species that often are not able to avoid high temperatures in their environment. Thus, it can be expected that adaptations to temperature/heat stress are frequent in nature. Furthermore heat stress shares characteristics with other stress factors, e.g., the type of cellular damage induced, and induces a suit of relatively well-studied molecular chaperones through the heat shock response, which are among the prime candidates conferring hormetic effects. Effects of exposure to stressful low temperatures show similarities to exposure to high temperatures as both induce cellular

[1]Genetics and Ecology, Department of Biological Sciences, University of Aarhus, Ny Munkegade, Building 1540, DK-8000 Aarhus C, Denmark.

[2]Department of Genetics and Biotechnology, University of Aarhus. P.O. Box 50, DK-8830 Tjele, Denmark

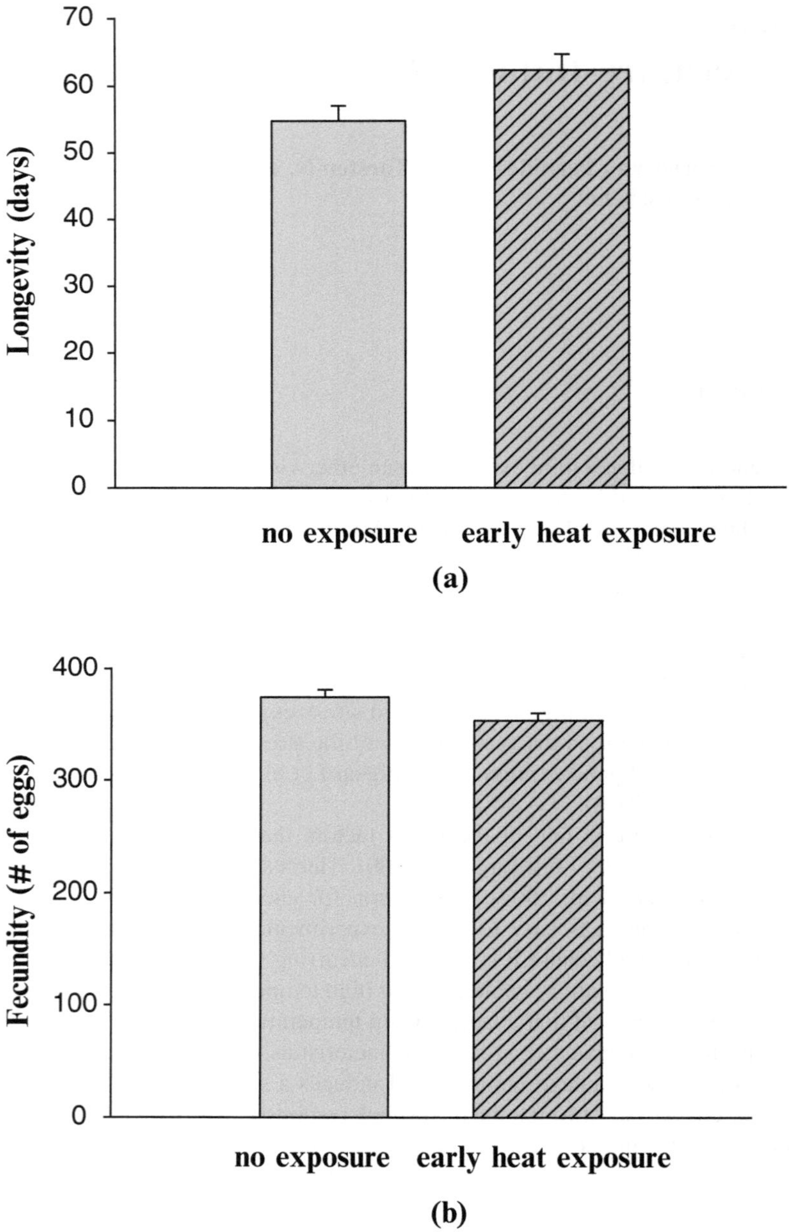

Fig. 1 Effects of repeated bouts of mild heat stress (34 °C for 3 h) applied at days 3, 6, 9 and 12 of adult *D. melanogaster* females on traits measured later in life. (a) longevity in days, (b) cumulative fecundity (days 2–18)

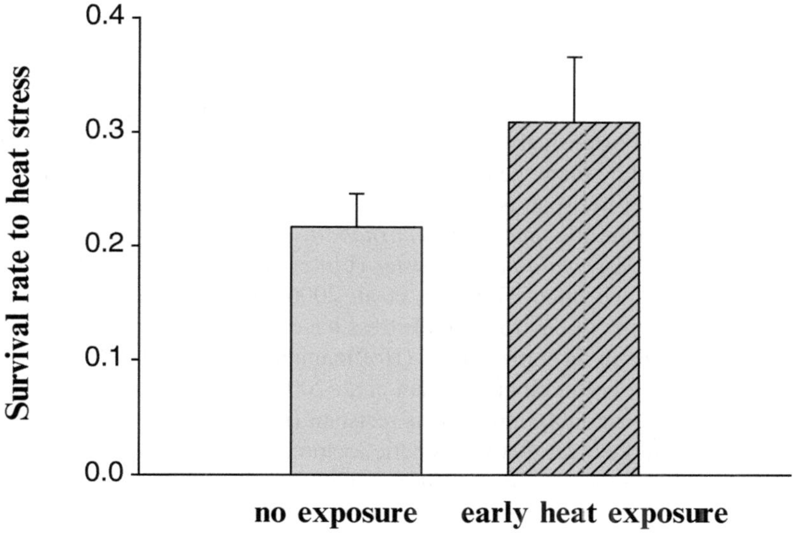

(c)

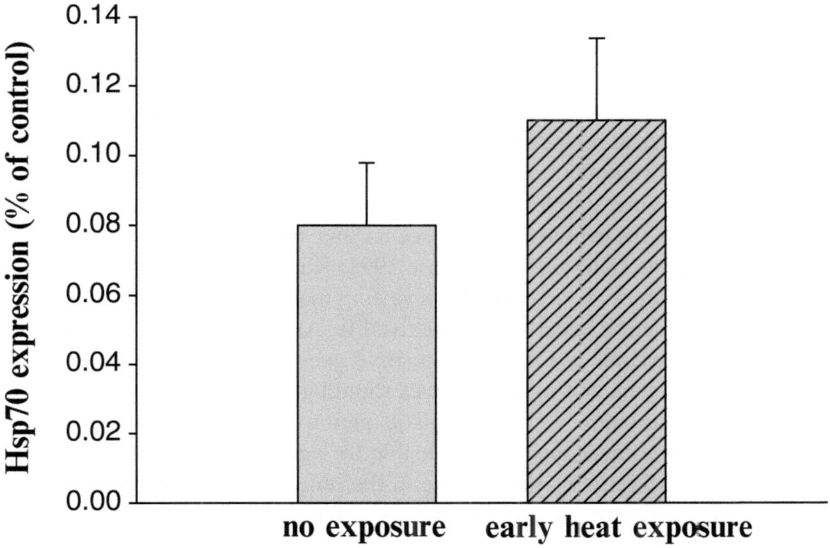

(d)

Fig. 1 (continued) (c) heat resistance at day 17 and (d) Hsp expression level after heat stress at day 17. The stress temperature and exposure time used to induce hormesis was chosen so that about one third of the maximal Hsp70 expression was induced (Redrawn from Hercus et al. 2003)

damage and stress responses that promote increased tolerance. Examples of cold-induced hormesis are rare but might have been overlooked (Le Bourg 2007).

Especially longevity has received attention in hormesis research partly because this trait has implications for medical research. The genetic background of life span has been investigated extensively in many species and is considered to be a quantitative trait influenced by many genes and by the environment. Detailed knowledge of the genetic basis of life span is still scarce even though several genes have been identified that modulate life span in *Caenorhabditis elegans* (Cypser et al. 2006; Broue et al. 2007), *Drosophila melanogaster* (Lin et al. 1998; Regina et al. 2000; Clancy et al. 2001) and mice (Boylston et al. 2006). Heat stress resistance and resistance to other types of environmental stress have been shown to be genetically correlated with longevity in some studies (Hoffmann and Parsons 1993; Norry and Loeschcke 2003), but not in others (Phelan et al. 2003). In addition, lines selected for long life are not invariably more stress resistant (Bubliy and Loeschcke 2005). Therefore, one would expect that the genetic architecture of longevity is complex and that many different genetic compositions can lead to a long life.

Evolutionary Theories and Mechanisms of Aging

From an evolutionary point of view there needs to be benefits associated with a trait for natural selection to operate on it, and this also apply for senescence. Most evolutionary theory revolves around trade offs between benefits and costs of different life-history strategies as resources are always limited. Investment of energy on maintaining life and on reproduction constitutes such a trade off. Either evolution will favor individuals to invest in longer life or in higher reproductive output. This is the trade off explaining the evolution of senescence and aging as stated in the disposable soma theory of aging (Kirkwood and Rose 1991; Kirkwood 2002). The theory suggests that highest fitness is achieved by investing mainly in maintenance and repair (soma) and reproduction in early reproductive life. At a given age (depending on the specific life-history strategy for the organism in question) little is gained by continued investment in soma and most resources should go into reproduction.

Mutation-accumulation and antagonistic pleiotropy are considered to be the evolutionary genetic mechanisms responsible for aging. The role of natural selection for viability decreases with age due to the reduced proportion that is alive at older age. For this reason, deleterious genetic effects that are expressed late in life will effectively not be selected against. As a result, mutations with late-age deleterious gene effects can accumulate in the genome. If the population is relieved of extrinsic mortality, these mutations become expressed and the soma will progressively deteriorate, i.e., it will show senescent ageing. This is the theory of mutation accumulation as stated by Medawar (1952). The theory of antagonistic pleiotropy of Williams (1957) is similar, but in addition states that genes can have pleiotropic effects in early and late life. Since the force of selection is weaker on late acting relative to early acting gene effects, mutations that have beneficial effects early in life can be selected for, even though they exert negative effects of similar magnitude later in life. As a consequence of such antagonistic gene effects, negative genetic correlations within and between life-history traits for their early and late effects will develop (Rose 1999; Vermeulen and Loeschcke 2007).

The Use of Model Organisms for Studying Hormesis and Aging

Even though the primary interest of hormesis research may be to understand the process of human ageing and possibly to increase the length of a healthy human life, progress will be greatly speeded up by studies utilizing animal models, which can provide faster and more accurate answers. Model organisms such as fruit flies (*D. melanogaster*), nematodes (*C. elegans*) and mice (*Mus musculus*) share many of the common features of complex systems of metazoan cells with humans, and therefore can complement human gerontological studies. Their strength lies in elucidating the impacts of environment and genes and their interactions for the phenotype in metazoan organisms, and thus be useful in identifying genes that influence life span and 'healthy aging' in humans.

D. melanogaster is well suited for many types of studies related to hormesis and aging research, because there is detailed knowledge of the embryonic development, behaviour and physiology of this species. Moreover, a suite of genetic techniques can be utilised. Some of these techniques have already been used to study both stress responses and aging (e.g., Nielsen et al. 2005; Baldal et al. 2006). The availability of a fully sequenced genome (Adams et al. 2000) allows the construction of gene expression arrays, including commercially available arrays containing approximately 13,000 genes. Although many of these genes are of unknown function such studies can provide knowledge of new genes and pathways involved in specific situations, and has been used to describe the genome wide gene expression response to various stresses (Girardot et al. 2004; Landis et al. 2004; Sørensen et al. 2005), aging and caloric restriction (Pletcher et al. 2002; Landis et al. 2004), selection for stress resistance (Sørensen et al. 2007a) and inbreeding (Kristensen et al. 2005) and genotype by environment interactions (Kristensen et al. 2006).

Hormesis – A Definition

Hormesis can be defined as 'stimulatory effect of low doses of substances or treatments known to be toxic or harmful at higher doses' (modified from Cypser et al. 2006). This extended definition is broad as it covers all possible factors or substances on all performance traits. All substances or environmental factors are predicted to have an optimum level for each organism in a given environment (Parsons 2003). Usually life span and resistance to the applied stress as well as other stresses are investigated. For some traits mild stress is only beneficial in some cases, while for other traits a hormetic effect is generally found. Thus, if several traits are measured without a strong hypothesis as to whether hormesis is expected results are difficult to interpret. We need to collect knowledge about mechanisms of life span determination and induction of hormesis to be able to figure out when, in which traits and under which conditions hormesis can be expected to occur.

Hormesis, Hardening and Acclimation

Hormesis is a general phenomenon that occurs across plant and animal species and is induced by multiple stress factors. The stress level inducing a strong hormetic effect varies but should be mild to prevent cells and organisms from suffering damage from the stress, but still strong enough to induce stress repair systems thought to be responsible for the hormetic effects. This level is expected to vary among rearing environments, stress types, species, sexes and populations. The hormetic window is expected to be quite narrow under many situations, thus, no or even negative effects could be expected to occur frequently.

In a sense hormesis can be regarded as a plastic response with similarity to hardening or acclimation, terms used in physiology to describe a short or long-term preconditioning to an environmental factor. Both hardening and acclimation to a mild or sub-lethal environmental stressor (e.g., low or high temperature) often leads to an increased performance with respect to later exposure to a more stressful environment (e.g., stressful temperatures). Similar, with respect to hormesis a mild environmental stress (e.g., high or low temperature) leads to increased performance later in life. However, when studying hormesis it is not performance with respect to a higher dose or stronger exposure that is measured but rather effects on other traits such as life span. With respect to hardening and acclimation "the beneficial acclimation hypothesis" states that acclimation is preparing the organism to a later treatment of the same kind but possibly more extreme, so that compared to non-acclimated individuals there should be an advantage of the acclimated individuals (Huey and Berrigan 1996; Huey et al. 1999). The net benefit depends on the costs of the acclimation treatment, and the costs may exceed the benefits (Loeschcke and Hoffmann 2002). A mild heat treatment can increase heat resistance for some days but with a cost on fecundity (Krebs and Loeschcke 1994). Similar when studying hormesis with respect to a fitness component or life-history trait, we study fitness in a laboratory environment that usually is benign – while evolution has shaped the fitness landscape and the involved trade-offs in a usually more stressful natural environment (Parsons 2000). The costs and benefits may partly be independent from each other and environment- and genotype-specific – as are hormetic effects of mild heat or cold temperature treatments.

Most organisms have plastic responses to environmental stress that ensure increased tolerance to similar types of stress in the future. Such plastic responses are expected to occur in natural populations as they will improve fitness in variable environments. The connection to longevity should probably not be looked for from an evolutionary adaptation perspective. Long life is not selected for or against in natural populations as most individuals tend to die of other causes before the onset of aging (for a review see Vermeulen and Loeschcke 2007). Thus, the observation that exposure to mild heat stress increases longevity and resistance to stress later in life does not necessarily mean that hormesis is important for evolution in biological systems. Firstly, due to the above-mentioned argument that selection does not operate at post reproductive lifespan and, secondly, because mild heat stress at a young age might affect reproduction negatively – thereby reducing fitness (Fig. 1b). Thus, if longevity is increased by stress exposures it is a side effect of the mechanism responding to the stress and ensuring stress resistance. Acclimation and hardening do however not fully explain hormesis. The terms are used to describe short-term benefits of, e.g., exposure to mild heat stress which increases resistance to more severe heat stress exposure. This benefit is normally of short duration and after a few days or hours the acclimation/hardening effect cannot be detected. With hormesis, however, a mild stress exposure at a young age has been shown to have lifelong benefits.

The Connection Between Hormesis, Stress Resistance and Longevity

Generally there seems to be a tendency for more stress resistant organisms to be long lived. However, long lived individuals are not always more resistant and if they are, often only to some stressors. Furthermore, the threshold level of specific stressors with the potential for extending life span or delay aging varies between experiments (Minois 2000; Norry and Loeschcke 2003; Landis et al. 2004; Wang et al. 2004; Bubliy and Loeschcke 2005). Thus, there is not a clear relationship between stress resistance and longevity, but is seems that "while stress resistance appears necessary for lifespan extension, it is not sufficient" (Cypser et al. 2006).

Even though increased life span and increased stress resistance usually are both induced by a hormetic treatment and, thus, seem to share stress inducible mechanisms (Minois 2000) this is not always the case. Some genes in the insulin-like signaling pathway play a large role for hormetically induced life extension in *C. elegans*, but only one of the three genes investigated was required for hormetically induced thermotolerance supporting the idea of partly separated mechanisms (Cypser et al. 2006).

Mechanisms Behind Temperature-Induced Hormesis

General Mechanisms

There are two main groups of biological explanations for heat-induced hormesis on life span. One is genes directly affecting life span. Here a few candidates have been identified in several species, but the connection to hormesis is not clear (but see Cypser et al. 2006). The other is genes and processes responding to (heat) stress. It is assumed that several factors from each category contribute to explaining hormesis although the contribution of various mechanisms is poorly understood. Stress responding genes involved in hormesis are thought to be found among the genes involved in various housekeeping systems induced by stress, including oxidative stress scavengers, DNA repair systems and the heat shock proteins (Hsps) (Rattan 2004). Even though inducible Hsps are prime candidates for contributing to the phenomenon of heat-induced hormesis, the experimental evidence is scarce.

Verbeke et al. (2001) showed that mild heat shocks have long-lasting beneficial effects on several traits in aging human skin fibroblasts. The treated cells showed a reduced accumulation of oxidized and glycoxidized proteins which normally is associated with age-related change (see the chapter "Hormetic modulation of aging in human cells"). These results suggest that the reduced amount of damaged proteins after mild heat stress was caused by an increased ability of the cells to cope with oxidative stress, and to synthesize Hsps responsible for protein capping and refolding (Verbeke et al. 2001; chapter "Hormetic modulation of aging in human cells"). Also Tatar et al. (1997) and Wang et al. (2004) have published results verifying that Hsps are one of the mechanisms explaining hormesis. They showed that overexpression of Hsp70, Hsp26 and Hsp27, respectively, leads to increased life span in *Drosophila*. However, an experiment using the same transgenic lines as Tatar et al. failed to detect any beneficial effect of Hsp70 overexpression on longevity (Minois et al. 2001).

The role of the heat response for hormetic effects has been studied using a mutant *D. melanogaster* line with a heat sensitive heat shock factor (Hsf). The mutant line carried a heat sensitive Hsf which is inactivated by heat stress while a rescued line was able to express the heat stress response (Jedlicka et al. 1997; Nielsen et al. 2005). The results showed that mild heat stress in early life led to increased heat resistance and longevity in males only, and only in the line able to express the functional Hsf after heat stress (i.e., the heat shock response) suggesting that Hsps are essential for heat-induced hormesis in longevity and for induced heat stress resistance at least in males (Sørensen et al. 2007). This study thus looked at the effect of deficiency of all Hsf inducible genes which could have some advantages over studies on single Hsps and overexpression. Hsps are considered important for all organisms at all times and the level of expression is tightly regulated to avoid the associated costs of expression (Sørensen et al. 2003). Overexpression of Hsps might lead to deleterious effects (Krebs and Loeschcke 1994; Krebs and Feder 1997; Feder and Hofmann 1999) and possible regulatory feed backs which might blur beneficial effects. Therefore, effects of deficiency might be more clearly observed.

Different Mechanisms in Males and Females?

Reports of sex-specific hormetic effects are common, and often beneficial effects of mild stress are larger in males. Hormetic effects of exposure to heat and hypergravity have been shown to be restricted to the male gender (Le Bourg et al. 2000; Minois 2000; Le Bourg et al. 2002; Sørensen et al. 2007). However, Le Bourg et al. (2001)

and Hercus et al. (2003) did find heat-induced hormesis on life span in female *D. melanogaster* when exposing young individuals to several mild heat treatments (Fig. 1a), suggesting that the phenomenon exists in both sexes, but that females have a different sensitivity and/or that hormesis is induced by partly different mechanisms in the two sexes. The authors also found that the hormetic effects disappeared or even became negative, when the mild heat treatments started at a slightly later age, showing that the net effect of costs and benefit functions had reversed (Hercus et al. 2003). A less dramatic decrease with age in the benefits from a mild heat shock has been found in *C. elegans* (Olsen et al. 2006). Differences in hormetic effects between males and females may be related to the fact that females in contrast to males have to trade off stress resistance and reproduction (see next section) (Salmon et al. 2001).

The Impact of Reproduction and Caloric Restrictions on Hormetic Effects

Sex dependent hormetic effects may relate to the reproductive status of the organisms. At least in *Drosophila* evidence suggests that life span of mated and virgin flies is very different. Vermeulen and Bijlsma (2006) showed that lines selected for virgin longevity without selecting for age at reproduction did show an increase in longevity of 21–38%, but no decrease in reproduction. However, longevity for mated individuals in these lines was not increased compared to the controls. Thus, the genetic mechanism determining mated and virgin life span is not necessarily identical.

Caloric restrictions can also have a big impact on longevity and therefore the nutritional status might influence on any study investigating hormesis. Restrictions on nutrient intake have been shown to slow down the process of aging in a range of organisms including yeast (Jiang et al. 2000), nematodes (Braeckman et al. 2001), *Drosophila* (Magwere et al. 2004) and rodents (Yu et al. 1985). Caloric restrictions have also been shown to reduce reproductive output and to retard the development of age-related diseases.

In many studies on hormesis the nutrient intake and reproductive status of the investigated individuals are not reported. Thus, it is not clear whether the effects of dietary restriction act through a hormesis-like mechanism or only directly in a trade off with reproduction. This is of concern and may explain some of the inconsistency of results on similar stress treatments and in similar organisms. Reduced reproduction in individuals exposed to mild (heat) stress (Fig. 1b) may be partly responsible for the hormetic effect on longevity and later exposure to severe stresses – again because more energy is invested in soma in mildly stressed individuals.

Cold-Induced Hormesis

Different types of stress might induce different mechanisms promoting hormesis. Hypergravity has successfully been applied to induce increased life span (see the chapter "Hypergravity in *Drosophila melanogaster*"). However, hypergravity does not induce Hsp70 expression, and flies exposed to hypergravity do not benefit from Hsp70 overexpression, although hypergravity induces thermotolerance in both overexpressing and control strains (Minois et al. 2001; Le Bourg et al. 2002; Minois and Vaynberg 2002). Furthermore, hypergravity, but not heat, has been shown to decrease the "behavioural aging", i.e., preserving the ability to maintain a higher climbing and locomotor activity at old age in flies (see the chapter "Hypergravity in *Drosophila melanogaster*").

One study has shown hormetic effects of low temperatures. Le Bourg (2007) exposed flies to repeated cold shocks and found hormesis on longevity, behavioural aging and both heat and cold shock resistance in aged flies. Like hypergravity the exposure to short-term cold shocks does not lead to a strong induction of Hsps (Overgaard et al. 2005). Another similarity between hypergravity and cold shock on the hormetic effect of these stimuli is that the stress has been applied over longer periods, either constant (hypergravity) or repeatedly (cold) over nearly 2 weeks of early life (Le Bourg et al. 2002; Le Bourg 2007). This is in contrast to heat where hormetic effects can be induced by relatively few (1–4) and short (few hours) bursts of stress (Le Bourg et al. 2001; Hercus et al. 2003; Kristensen et al. 2003; Sørensen et al. 2007). The effect of cold exposure on the hormetic effect thus resembles exposure to hypergravity more so than heat exposure. It is possible that the potential for cold-induced hormesis is still rather unexplored as cold acclimation and cold hardening responses are common (Hoffmann et al. 2003). These responses increase cold resistance and thus possibly might show hormesis under the right conditions. The lack of reports on cold-induced hormesis might be explained by the relative long-term and repeated treatments that seem to be necessary to induce hormesis by cold temperatures (Le Bourg 2007).

Despite that hypergravity and cold apparently are not associated with Hsps they cannot be considered independently of Hsps. Even though hypergravity itself does not induce Hsp70, flies showing hormesis due to hypergravity also express more Hsp70 when heat stressed compared to controls (Minois et al. 1999; Le Bourg et al. 2002). It is unclear what this increased expression of Hsps means. However, it could be regarded as indicating an increased sensitivity/responsiveness in hormetic organisms – even if the stress inducing hormesis does not itself induce Hsps.

Thus, Hsps seem to play some role for heat-induced hormesis while the importance of Hsps for hormesis induced by cold and other stresses is not clear and hormesis seems to be caused by a suit of mechanisms of which some are shared among stress types and some are stress-specific.

Perspectives

During the last century we have seen a dramatic increase in the average expected life span of humans in most parts of the world. This increase has mainly been due to environmental effects such as better nutrition, housing and improvements in modern medicine; in other words we have eliminated much of the physical stress earlier experienced by humans in the industrial parts of the world. However, as the increase in longevity has been less dramatic during the last decades, further increases in life span and, even more important, of good health late in life, will probably be grounded by a better understanding of the genetics behind aging and age-related diseases.

Evolutionary expectations predict that overall fitness should not be improved by applying stress to natural organisms (Forbes 2000). However, the hormesis phenomenon might still be relevant for single traits like life span or healthy aging and especially in humans or domesticated animals and plants that live in artificially benign environments, where natural selection and stress levels are reduced during early life.

Thus, hormesis seems to be a complex phenomenon that is the sum of multiple mechanisms, which are difficult to separate as they are all induced by stress. Surely, several mechanisms seem to contribute to the net effects as different stress treatments affect different traits such as life span, mortality rate, behavioural aging and several types of stress resistance differently. Furthermore, the exact application of the stress (e.g., timing, strength and duration) is crucial for the outcome of the treatment. In addition to this, as males and females and virgins and mated individuals seem to have different sensitivity to hormesis induction, the timing, strength and duration that may fit to induce hormesis in one gender may not do so in the other. Also caloric intake and nutrient balance interact with the hormetic effects of temperature, hypergravity and other types of stimuli. Therefore there is an urgent need for timely designed experiments controlling for all those factors that may explain non-consistency of results obtained so far.

There is still a lot we need to know in more detail before therapeutic application of (temperature) hormesis can be utilized. To do the type of research needed in humans there are several practical and ethical problems that make the use of model organisms such as *Drosophila* ideal. The hypotheses generated by these investigations can then at a later stage be applied to other organisms including humans.

At present we need to investigate mechanisms and changes induced in aging organisms and the changes that take place (or that do not take place) due to hormesis. We need to identify and understand the trade offs involved, e.g., between life span and reproduction and the assumed costs of the stress inductions. One place for advancement is to take advantage of the molecular technological developments and utilize studies of protein expression, metabolites and single nucleotide polymorphisms (SNPs) and whole genome gene expression patterns by micro arrays (Pletcher et al. 2002) that become available for model organisms.

A large task is to develop methods to estimate or measure the stress perceived by an organism. Not only the stress perceived at any given time, but more difficult also the accumulated level of different stress exposures throughout the life of an individual, that means its specific history of stress exposure throughout life. This is important if we want to use hormesis as a therapeutic treatment in humans, as studies have shown that the appropriate level of stress may depend on both the genetic background as well as the environment of the organism. Too high levels of stress will lead to damaging effects and thus potentially decreased life span. To apply hormetic treatments as a therapy, one needs to develop methods of measuring the individual stress history and predicting the appropriate hormetic dose needed on an individual basis.

Acknowledgements We are grateful to Corneel Vermeulen, Eric Le Bourg and Suresh Rattan for helpful comments on earlier versions of the ms, to the Danish Research Councils for support through post doctoral fellowships (JGS and TNK) and frame and centre grants (VL) as well as to the Lundbeck and Carlsberg Foundations for a post doctoral fellowship to PS.

References

Adams MD, Celniker SE, Holt RA, Evans CA, Gocayne JD, Amanatides PG, Scherer SE, Li PW, Hoskins RA, Galle RF, George RA, Lewis SE and Richards S (2000) The genome sequence of *Drosophila melanogaster*. Science 287:2185–2195

Baldal EA, Baktawar W, Brakefield PM and Zwaan BJ (2006) Methuselah life history in a variety of conditions, implications for the use of mutants in longevity research. Exp Gerontol 41:1126–1135

Boylston WH, DeFord JH and Papaconstantinou J (2006) Identification of longevity-associated genes in long-lived Snell and Ames dwarf mice. Age 28:125–144

Braeckman BP, Houthoofd K and Vanfleteren JR (2001) Insulin-like signaling, metabolism, stress resistance and aging in *Caenorhabditis elegans*. Mech Age Dev 122:673–693

Broue F, Liere P, Kenyon C and Baulieu EE (2007) A steroid hormone that extends the lifespan of *Caenorhabditis elegans*. Aging Cell 6:87–94

Bubliy OA, Imasheva AG and Loeschcke V (1998) Selection for knockdown resistance to heat in *Drosophila melanogaster* at high and low larval densities. Evolution 52:619–625

Bubliy OA and Loeschcke V (2005) Correlated responses to selection for stress resistance and longevity in a laboratory population of *Drosophila melanogaster*. J Evol Biol 18:789–803

Clancy DJ, Gems D, Harshman LG, Oldham S, Stocker H, Hafen E, Leevers SJ and Partridge L (2001) Extension of life-span by loss of CHICO, a *Drosophila* insulin receptor substrate protein. Science 292:104–106

Cypser JR, Tedesco P and Johnson TE (2006) Hormesis and aging in *Caenorhabditis elegans*. Exp Gerontol 41:935–939

Dahlgaard J, Loeschcke V, Michalak P and Justesen J (1998) Induced thermotolerance and associated expression of the heat-shock protein Hsp70 in adult *Drosophila melanogaster*. Funct Ecol 12:786–793

Feder ME and Hofmann GE (1999) Heat-shock proteins, molecular chaperones, and the stress response: Evolutionary and ecological physiology. Annu Rev Physiol 61:243–282

Forbes VE (2000) Is hormesis an evolutionary expectation? Funct Ecol 14:12–24

Girardot F, Monnier V and Tricoire H (2004) Genome wide analysis of common and specific stress responses in adult *Drosophila melanogaster*. Bmc Genomics 5:74

Hercus MJ, Loeschcke V and Rattan SIS (2003) Lifespan extension of *Drosophila melanogaster* through hormesis by repeated mild heat stress. Biogerontology 4:149–156

Hoffmann AA and Parsons PA (1993) Selection for adult desiccation resistance in *Drosophila melanogaster* – fitness components, larval resistance and stress correlations. Biol J Linn Soc 48:43–54

Hoffmann AA, Sørensen JG and Loeschcke V (2003) Adaptation of *Drosophila* to temperature extremes: bringing together quantitative and molecular approaches. J Therm Biol 28:175–216

Huey RB, Berrigan D, Gilchrist GW and Herron JC (1999) Testing the adaptive significance of acclimation: A strong inference approach. Am Zool 39:323–336

Huey RB and Berrigan DA (1996) Testing evolutionary hypothesis of acclimation. In: IA Johnston and AF Bennett (Eds.) Animals and Temperature: Phenotypic and Evolutionary Adaptation. Cambridge University Press, Cambridge

Jedlicka P, Mortin MA and Wu C (1997) Multiple functions of *Drosophila* heat shock transcription factor in vivo. Embo J 16:2452–2462

Jiang JC, Jaruga E, Repnevskaya MV and Jazwinski SM (2000) An intervention resembling caloric restriction prolongs life span and retards aging in yeast. FASEB J 14 2135–2137

Khazaeli AA, Tatar M, Pletcher SD and Curtsinger JW (1997) Heat-induced longevity extension in *Drosophila*. I. Heat treatment, mortality, and thermotolerance. J Gerontol 52A:B48–B52

Kirkwood TBL (2002) Evolution of ageing. Mech Ageing Dev 123:737–745

Kirkwood TBL and Rose MR (1991) Evolution of senescence – Late survival sacrificed for reproduction. Philos T Roy Soc B 332:15–24

Krebs RA and Feder ME (1997) Deleterious consequences of Hsp70 overexpression in *Drosophila melanogaster* larvae. Cell Stress Chaperon 2:60–71

Krebs RA and Loeschcke V (1994) Costs and benefits of activation of the heat-shock response in *Drosophila melanogaster*. Funct Ecol 8:730–737

Kristensen TN, Sørensen JG and Loeschcke V (2003) Mild heat stress at a young age in *Drosophila melanogaster* leads to increased Hsp70 synthesis after stress exposure later in life. J Genet 82:89–94

Kristensen TN, Sorensen P, Kruhoffer M, Pedersen KS and Loeschcke V (2005) Genome-wide analysis on inbreeding effects on gene expression in *Drosophila melanogaster*. Genetics 171:157–167

Kristensen TN, Sørensen P, Pedersen KS, Kruhøffer M and Loeschcke V (2006) Inbreeding by environmental interactions affect gene expression in *Drosophila melanogaster*. Genetics 173:1329–1336

Landis GN, Abdueva D, Skvortsov D, Yang JD, Rabin BE, Carrick J, Tavare S and Tower J (2004) Similar gene expression patterns characterize aging and oxidative stress in *Drosophila melanogaster*. P Natl Acad Sci USA 101:7663–7668

Le Bourg E (2007) Hormetic effects of repeated exposures to cold at young age on longevity, aging and resistance to heat or cold shocks in *Drosophila melanogaster*. Biogerontology 8:431–444

Le Bourg E and Minois N (1997) Increased longevity and resistance to heat shock in *Drosophila melanogaster* flies exposed to hypergravity. C R Acad Sci, Sér 3, Sci. Vie 320:215–221

Le Bourg E and Minois N (1999) A mild stress, hypergravity exposure, postpones behavioral aging in *Drosophila melanogaster*. Exp Gerontol 34:157–172

Le Bourg E, Minois N, Bullens P and Baret P (2000) A mild stress due to hypergravity exposure at young age increases longevity in *Drosophila melanogaster* males. Biogerontology 1:145–155

Le Bourg E, Valenti P, Lucchetta P and Payre F (2001) Effects of mild heat shocks at young age on aging and longevity in *Drosophila melanogaster*. Biogerontology 2:155–164

Le Bourg E, Valenti P and Payre F (2002) Lack of hypergravity-associated longevity extension in *Drosophila melanogaster* flies overexpressing hsp70. Biogerontology 3:355–364

Lin YJ, Seroude L and Benzer S (1998) Extended life-span and stress resistance in the *Drosophila* mutant Methuselah. Science 282:934–946

Loeschcke V and Hoffmann AA (2002) The detrimental acclimation hypothesis Trends Ecol Evol 17:407–408

Magwere T, Chapman T and Partridge L (2004) Sex differences in the effect of dietary restriction on life span and mortality rates in female and male *Drosophila melanogaster*. J Gerontol, Ser A-Biol Sci Med Sci 59:3–9

Malmendal A, Overgaard J, Bundy JG, Sørensen JG, Nielsen NC, Loeschcke V and Holmstrup M (2006) Metabolomic profiling of heat stress: hardening and recovery of homeostasis in *Drosophila*. Am J Physiol-Reg I 291:R205–R212

Medawar PB (1952) An Unsolved Problem in Biology. H. K. Lewis, London

Minois N (2000) Longevity and aging: beneficial, effects of exposure to mild stress. Biogerontology 1:15–29

Minois N, Guinaudy MJ, Payre F and Le Bourg E (1999) Hsp70 induction may explain the long-lasting resistance to heat of *Drosophila melanogaster* having lived in hypergravity. Mech Age Dev 109:65–77

Minois N, Khazaeli AA and Curtsinger JW (2001) Locomotor activity as a function of age and life span in *Drosophila melanogaster* overexpressing hsp70. Exp Gerontol 36:1137–1153

Minois N and Vaynberg S (2002) Fecundity and life span in transgenic *Drosophila melanogaster* overexpressing hsp70. Biogerontology 3:301–306

Nielsen MM, Overgaard J, Sørensen JG, Holmstrup M, Justesen J and Loeschcke V (2005) Role of the heat-shock factor during heat and cold hardening and for the resistance to severe heat and cold stress. J Insect Physiol 51:1320–1329

Norry FM and Loeschcke V (2003) Heat-induced expression of a molecular chaperone decreases by selecting for long-lived individuals. Exp Gerontol 38:673–681

Olsen A, Vantipalli MC, Walker GA and Lithgow GJ (2006) Checkpoint proteins determine organismal stress resistance and lifespan in *C. elegans*. Toxicology 226:18

Overgaard J, Sørensen JG, Petersen SO, Loeschcke V and Holmstrup M (2005) Changes in membrane lipid composition following rapid cold hardening in *Drosophila melanogaster*. J Insect Physiol 51:1173–1182

Parsons PA (2000) Hormesis: an adaptive expectation with emphasis on ionizing radiation. J Appl Toxicol 20:103–112

Parsons PA (2003) From the stress theory of aging to energetic and evolutionary expectations for longevity. Biogerontology 4:63–73

Phelan JP, Archer MA, Beckman KA, Chippindale AK, Nusbaum TJ and Rose MR (2003) Breakdown in correlations during laboratory evolution. I. Comparative analyses of *Drosophila* populations. Evolution 57:527–535

Pletcher SD, Macdonald SJ, Marguerie R, Certa U, Stearns SC, Goldstein DB and Partridge L (2002) Genome-wide transcript profiles in aging and calorically restricted *Drosophila melanogaster*. Curr Biol 12:712–723

Rattan SIS (1998) Repeated mild heat shock delays ageing in cultured human skin fibroblasts. Biochem Mol Biol Int 45:753–760

Rattan SIS (2004) Aging intervention, prevention, and therapy through hormesis. J Gerontol a-Biol 59:B705–B709

Regina B, Reenan RA, Nilsen SP and Helfand SL (2000) Extended life-span conferred by cotransporter gene mutations in *Drosophila*. Science 290:2137–2140

Rose MR (1999) Genetics of aging in *Drosophila*. Exp Gerontol 34:577–585

Salmon AB, Marx DB and Harshman LG (2001) A cost of reproduction in *Drosophila melanogaster*: Stress susceptibility. Evolution 55:1600–1608

Scannapieco AC, Sørensen JG, Loeschcke V and Norry FM (2007) Heat-induced hormesis in longevity of two sibling *Drosophila* species. Biogerontology 8:315–325

Sørensen JG, Kristensen TN and Loeschcke V (2003) The evolutionary and ecological role of heat shock proteins. Ecol Lett 6:1025–1037

Sørensen JG, Kristensen TN, Kristensen KV and Loeschcke V (2007b). Sex specific effects of heat induced in Hsf-deficient *Drosophila melanogaster*. Exp Gerontol 42: 1123–1129. doi:10.1016/j.exger.2007.09.001

Sørensen JG, Nielsen MM, Kruhøffer M, Justesen J and Loeschcke V (2005) Gene profile analysis of the temporal heat stress response in *Drosophila melanogaster*. Cell Stress Chaperon 10:312–328

Sørensen JG, Nielsen MM and Loeschcke V (2007a) Gene expression profile analysis of *Drosophila melanogaster* selected for resistance to environmental stressors. J Evolution Biol 20:1624–1636

Tatar M, Khazaeli AA and Curtsinger JW (1997) Chaperoning extended life. Nature 390:30

Verbeke P, Clark BFC and Rattan SIS (2001) Reduced levels of oxidized and glycoxidized proteins in human fibroblasts exposed to repeated mild heat shock during serial passaging in vitro. Free Radical Bio Med 31:1593–1602

Vermeulen CJ and Bijlsma R (2006) Changes in genetic architecture during relaxation in *Drosophila melanogaster* selected on divergent virgin life span. J Evol Biol 19:216–227
Vermeulen CJ and Loeschcke V (2007) Longevity and the stress response in *Drosophila*. Exp Gerontol 42:153–159
Wang HD, Kazemi-Esfarjani P and Benzer S (2004) Multiple-stress analysis for isolation of *Drosophila* longevity genes. P Natl Acad Sci USA 101:12610–12615
Williams GC (1957) Pleiotropy, natural selection, and the evolution of senescence. Evolution 11:398–411
Yu BP, Masoro EJ and McMahan CA (1985) Nutritional influences on aging of Fischer-344 Rats.1. Physical, metabolic, and longevity characteristics. J Gerontol 40:657–670

Chapter 6
Hormetic Modulation of Aging in Human Cells

Suresh I.S. Rattan

Introduction

An experimental model system that has been used in testing and applying hormesis as a modulator of aging is the so-called Hayflick system of cellular aging *in vitro*. In modern biogerontology, the terms "cellular aging", "cell senescence" or "replicative senescence" imply the study of normal diploid cells in culture, which during serial subcultivation undergo a multitude of changes culminating in the irreversible cessation of cell division. This process of cellular aging or replicative senescence *in vitro* is commonly known as the Hayflick phenomenon, and the limited division potential of normal cells is called the Hayflick limit, in recognition of the observations first reported by Leonard Hayflick in 1961. In many organisms, several cell types retain the capacity to divide during most of the adult lifespan, and are required to divide repeatedly or infrequently in carrying out various functions of the body. These functions include the immune response, blood formation, bone formation, and repair and regeneration of various tissues. Epithelial cells, epidermal basal cells (keratinocytes), fibroblasts, osteoblasts, myoblasts, glial cells and lymphocytes constitute major differentiated and proliferating cell types of an organism, and are distinct from the pluripotent stem cells. It is not only their differentiated and specialized functions that are critical for the organism, their capacity to divide is an integral part of their role in organismic growth, development, maintenance and survival (for details on the aging *in vitro* of various cell types (see Kaul and Wadhwa 2003).

The study of age-related changes in the physiology, biochemistry and molecular biology of isolated cell populations has greatly expanded our understanding of the fundamental aspects of aging. In addition to the normal diploid fibroblasts which

Laboratory of Cellular Ageing, Department of Molecular Biology, University of Aarhus, DK-8000 Aarhus C, Denmark.

Address for correspondence:
Dr. Suresh I.S. Rattan, Department of Molecular Biology, University of Aarhus, Gustav Wieds Vej 10C, DK-8000 Aarhus C, Denmark. Phone: +45 8942 5034; Fax: +45 8612 3178; e-mail: rattan@mb.au.dk

E. Le Bourg and S.I.S. Rattan (eds.), *Mild Stress and Healthy Aging.*

have been the most frequently used cells for studies on cellular ageing *in vitro*, a variety of other cell types including epithelial cells, endothelial cells, keratinocytes, glial cells, lymphocytes and osteoblasts have also been used. Although the exact culturing conditions (such as the type of the culture medium, the source of growth factors, the use of antibiotics, and the incubation temperature, humidity and gaseous composition) may vary for different cell types, serial subcultivation or serial passaging of normal diploid differentiated cells can be performed only a limited number of time. The cumulative number of cell proliferations, measured as the cumulative population doubling level achieved *in vitro*, depends upon several biological factors, such as the maximum lifespan of the species, the age of the donor of the tissue biopsy, and the site of the biopsy. This is in contrast to the high proliferative capacity of transformed, cancerous and immortalized cells whose cultures can be subcultivated and maintained indefinitely.

Serial subcultivation of normal cells is accompanied by a progressive accumulation of a wide variety of changes before the final cessation of cell replication occurs. The progressively emerging senescent phenotype of serially passaged normal diploid cells can be categorized into the structural, physiological, and biochemical and molecular phenotypes, which can be used as biomarkers of cellular aging *in vitro*. Table 1 gives a summary of the major changes occurring during serial passaging and replicative senescence. For specific details for different cell types (see Kaul and Wadhwa 2003).

What is clear is that the development and use of the Hayflick system has been instrumental in creating a strong foundation for understanding the cellular and molecular basis of aging (Rattan 2003). Based on these studies, aging can be characterized as: (i) a progressive accumulation of macromolecular damage and increased molecular heterogeneity; and (ii) progressive shrinkage of the homeostatic/homeodynamic space due to the failure of maintenance and repair systems leading to increased vulnerability, diseases and eventual death (Rattan 2006). Application of hormesis as a modulator of aging in human cells is based in the

Table 1 Main categories of phenotypic changes occurring during cellular aging *in vitro*

1. *Structural phenotype*: Increase in cell size; change of shape from thin, long and spindle-like to flattened and irregular; loss of fingerprint-like arrangement in parallel arrays; increased number of vacuoles and dense lysosomal residual bodies containing UV-fluorescent pigments; rod-like polymerization of the cytoskeletal actin filaments and disorganized microtubules; and increased level of chromosomal aberrations and multinucleation.
2. *Physiological phenotype*: Reduced response to growth factors and other mitogens; increased sensitivity to toxins, drugs, irradiation and other stress; altered calcium flux, pH, viscosity and membrane potential; reduced respiration and energy metabolism; and increased duration of G1 phase of the cell cycle.
3. *Biochemical and molecular phenotype*: Decreased activity, specificity and fidelity of various enzymes; accumulation of post-translationally modified and inactivated proteins; reduced rates of protein synthesis and degradation; increased levels of oxidative damage in nuclear and mitochondrial DNA; reduced levels of methylated cytosines; reduced length of telomeres; and altered (increased or decreased) expression of several genes, including cell cycle check point genes.

above understanding of biological aging as a progressive failure of homeodynamics (Rattan 2001, 2004, 2006).

Mild Heat Shock-Induced Hormesis in Human Cells

High temperature stress is a widely used hormetic agent, not only because it is relatively easy to implement, but also because heat stress mainly acts through an evolutionarily highly conserved stress response pathway known as the heat shock (HS) response. HS response is one of the primordial intracellular defence mechanisms against stressful conditions in which extracellular stress, and intracellular stress from denatured proteins, initiates a series of events starting with signal transduction, activation and nuclear translocation of heat shock factors (HSF), DNA binding of HSF, preferential initiation of HS gene transcription, and preferential translation of heat shock proteins (HSP), which then perform various biological functions (Verbeke et al. 2001; Park et al. 2005). (*HS-induced hormesis in other aging organisms is discussed in other chapters in this book*).

In our labs, we have been testing the hormesis hypothesis of the beneficial effects of mild HS on the Hayflick system of cellular aging of normal human cells in culture. The mild HS conditions were selected from a series of pilot studies performed on testing the effects of 1 h HS at different temperatures, ranging from 37 °C to 45 °C, on the synthesis of HSP70 in the following 3 h period. Maximum HSP70 synthesis (more than eightfold synthesis as compared with that at 37 °C) was observed at 43 °C. However, at 41 °C, HS response was about one third of the maximum response, and so this temperature was selected for long-term studies in which the cells were exposed repeatedly to HS. Temperatures higher than 43 °C could not be used for repeated exposures.

Using a mild stress regimen of exposing serially passaged human adult skin fibroblasts to 41 °C for 1 h twice a week throughout their replicative lifespan *in vitro*, we have reported a wide variety of biological effects. A summary of our observations on the hormetic effects of repeated mild HS on human skin fibroblasts undergoing aging *in vitro* is given in Table 2.

We have also undertaken studies on the hormetic effects of repeated mild HS on normal human epidermal keratinocytes (NHEK), and the results obtained are very much similar to those for dermal fibroblasts (Rattan and Ali 2007). As previously observed for human skin fibroblasts, NHEK also showed a variety of cellular and biochemical hormetic anti-aging effects on repeated exposure to mild HS at 41 °C. These effects included maintenance of youthful cellular morphology, enhanced replicative lifespan, enhanced proteasomal activity, and increased levels of HSP (Rattan and Ali 2007). Additionally, we have also studied the effects of HS on Na, K-ATPase or the sodium pump. Mild HS significantly increased the content and activity of the pump in NHEK. However, the molecular mechanisms and interactions which bring about the mild HS-induced increase in the amounts and activity of Na, K-ATPase, and its consequences on other biochemical pathways, in NHEK

Table 2 Hormetic effects of repeated mild heat shock on human skin fibroblasts undergoing aging *in vitro*

Characteristic	Hormetic effect	Reference
Cell size	Reduced enlargement	Rattan 1998
Cellular morphology	Reduced irregularisation	Rattan 1998
Replicative lifespan	10–20% increase	Nielsen et al. 2006
Glycation, furasine level	50–80% reduction	Verbeke et al. 2001
Glycoxidation level	10–30% reduction	Verbeke et al. 2001
CML-rich protein level	20–85% reduction	Verbeke et al. 2001
Lipofuscin pigment level	6–29% reduction	Verbeke et al. 2001
Protein carbonyl levels	5–40% reduction	Verbeke et al. 2001
Reduced glutathione level	Threefold increase	Verbeke et al. 2001
Oxidised glutathione level	Twofold reduction	Verbeke et al. 2001
Induction of sugar-induced protein damage	Tenfold reduction	Verbeke et al. 2002
H_2O_2 decomposing ability	50–140% increase	Fonager et al. 2002
Survival after H_2O_2 exposure	10–18% increase	Fonager et al. 2002
Survival after ethanol exposure	10–40% increase	Fonager et al. 2002
Survival after UVA exposure	5–17% increase	Fonager et al. 2002
Hsp27 level	20–40% increase	Fonager et al. 2002
Hsc70 level	20% increase	Fonager et al. 2002
Hsp70 level	7–20-fold increase	Fonager et al. 2002
Hsp90 level	50–80% reduction	Fonager et al. 2002
Proteasome activities	40–90% increase	Beedholm et al. 2004
20S proteasome content	No change	Beedholm et al. 2004
19S activator content	No change	Beedholm et al. 2004
11S activator content	Increase	Beedholm et al. 2004
11S activator binding	Increase	Beedholm et al. 2004
Proteasomal oscillation	Enhanced stability	Kraft et al. 2006

during aging are yet to be elucidated. Notably, comparable hormetic effects could not be seen in NHEK repeatedly exposed to 43 °C, which underlines the differences between the beneficial effects of mild stress and the harmful effects of severe stress. Other hormetic effects of mild HS on NHEK include increased differentiation of keratinocytes in the presence of calcium, and reduced cytotoxic effects of glucose and glyoxal (Berge et al. 2007).

Other cell types in which we have initiated studies on the hormetic effects of mild HS are telomerase-immortalised human bone marrow stem cells, and human microvascular endothelial cells. In a pilot study we have reported that vitamin-D-induced differentiation of telomerase-immortalised bone marrow stem cells into osteoblasts could be enhanced by pre-exposure to mild HS (Nørgaard et al. 2006). Our more recent studies indicate that mild HS also promotes angiogenesis (measured by the tube formation assays) in human microvascular endothelial cells, and may stimulate the migration of human skin fibroblasts in a wound healing assay *in vitro* (*unpublished observations*). Further studies are in progress to unravel the molecular details of enhanced angiogenesis by endothelial cells and enhanced wound healing by fibroblasts exposed to single or multiple rounds of mild HS.

Possible Mechanisms of Hormetic Effects of Heat Stress

The possible pathways for the hormetic effects of repeated mild HS in human cells include an increase in the activities of the proteasome, increased levels of various HSP, and increased antioxidative enzyme activities, (Fonager et al. 2002; Beedholm et al. 2004). Furthermore, we have also shown that repeated mild HS at 41 °C, but not the severe HS at 42 °C, increased the replicative lifespan, and elevated and maintained the basal levels of MAP kinases JNK1, JNK2 and p38 in human skin fibroblasts (Nielsen et al. 2006).

Although the general mechanisms of severe HS response are well understood (Feder and Hofmann 1999; Verbeke et al. 2001; Sun and MacRae 2005), it is not clear whether there are any significant differences between mild HS which has hormetic effects, and severe HS, repeated exposure to which has deleterious effects (Park et al. 2005). It is likely that the physiological cost of stress in terms of energy utilisation, molecular damage overload and metabolic shift determine the difference between the outcome of mild and severe stress (Salvioli et al. 2001). Also, it is yet to be understood how the transient appearance of HSP leads to biologically amplified hormetic effects at various other levels of cellular functioning, such as improved proteasome activity, enhanced resistance to other stresses, maintenance of the cytoskeletal integrity and others.

Optimal HS response in terms of HSP synthesis and activity is essential for cell survival. In contrast, inefficient and altered HS response has been implicated in abnormal growth and development, aging and apoptosis (Söti et al. 2005; Verbeke et al. 2001). When a cell encounters a "stressor", modifications of the cytoskeleton, cytoplasmic structures, cell surface morphology, cellular redox status, DNA synthesis, protein metabolism and protein stability occur. Heat stress generates molecular damage, especially abnormally folded proteins, which can aggregate and initiate a sequence of stress response. The cellular stress response can be viewed as an adaptive response for the defence and maintenance of its structural and functional integrity.

Signaling pathways in HS: Signaling pathways involved in HS response are still largely unknown. However, some kinases in the stress pathways, such as stress activated protein kinase (SAPK) c-Jun terminal kinase (JNK or SAPK1) and p38 (SAPK2), are suggested to play an important role. HS activates within minutes the major signaling pathways involving mitogen-activated protein kinase (MAPK), extracellular signal-regulated kinase (ERK) and SAPK (Gabai et al. 1998; Dorion and Landry 2002). These kinases are involved in both survival and death pathways in response to other stresses and may, therefore, contribute significantly to the HS response (Gabai and Sherman 2002). Activation of p38 occurs very early during stress and leads to the phosphorylation of HSP27. It is triggered by a highly specific HS sensing pathway and requires the activation of upstream kinases such as the MAPKK MKK3/6 and the MAPKKK apoptosis signal-regulating kinase-1 (ASK1) (Meriin et al. 1999). HS is also thought to activate (and thus phosphorylate) the epidermal growth factor (EGF) receptor in an agonist-independent way (Dorion and Landry 2002). HS has also been shown to phosphorylate constitutive nitric oxide synthase at tyrosine residues and increase fas/CD95 expression on the cell membrane (Kiang et al. 2003). HS also increases the levels of calcium, sodium, cAMP, and inositol 1,4,5-trisphosphate (Kiang and Tsokos 1998).

It is suggested that JNK is preferentially associated with the protective effects of HS against severe stress (Park and Liu 2001). A major mechanism for HS-induced JNK appears to be the direct inhibition of the JNK phosphatase that normally inactivates JNK. In the absence of this phosphatase, the basal activity of MAPKK4 (MKK4) is sufficient to activate JNK (Meriin et al. 1999). An early and transient activation of the JNK and p38 pathways is usually associated with survival and differentiation, whereas a late and sustained activation might point to apoptosis (Dorion and Landry 2002). Therefore a balance between the JNK and p38 pathways (apoptotic) and ERK pathways (survival), and their interplay, determine whether a cell exposed to HS will die or survive and become stress tolerant (Gabai and Sherman 2002). We have observed a rapid activation of MAP-kinases in terms of phosphorylation after 41 °C or 42 °C HS, and cells exposed to multiple rounds of 41 °C or 42 °C HS seem to have an increased amount of total JNK and p38 as compared with unstressed cells (Nielsen et al. 2006).

Activation of heat shock factors: The induction of the HS response is facilitated through the HSF working as molecular links between environmental stresses and the stress response (Kiang and Tsokos 1998; Verbeke et al. 2001). The four vertebrate HSF are expressed constitutively and cooperate functionally. HSF1 is a long-lived protein, it is an inactive monomer considered to be a general stress responsive factor which is expressed ubiquitously and is activated by mild HS as well as multiple environmental or physiological stresses. HSF2 is a short-lived protein present as an inactive dimer refractory to typical stress stimuli except proteasome inhibitors and is considered to be important during embryogenesis and spermatogenesis. HSF3 is also an inactive dimer and an important co-regulator of HSF1, activated by severe HS and chemical stress. HSF3 may exhibit complex interactions with other transcription factors governing development, growth and apoptosis, such as c-Myc and p53. HSF4 constitutively binds DNA even in non-stressed cells and is preferentially expressed in muscle, brain and pancreas (Verbeke et al. 2001).

In unstressed cells, HSF1 is both located in the cytoplasm and in the nucleus. It is maintained as a non DNA-binding inactive complex both by internal coiled-coil interactions and by stoichiometric binding with HSP90, HSP70 and other chaperones. The synergistic interaction between these chaperones modulates HSF1 activity by feedback repression (Shamovsky and Gershon 2004). During and after stress, the cellular proteins undergo denaturation and/or polyubiquitination and sequester the chaperones capping HSF1. The inactive HSF1 becomes free and translocates into the nucleus. HSF have a nuclear localization sequence that is both necessary for the transition of HSF from inactive to active state and for nuclear import. HSF1 is activated by trimerization and subsequent phosphorylation (Kiang and Tsokos 1998). Using electrophoretic mobility shift assay, we have demonstrated that RMHS at 41 °C activates HSF1 and facilitates its nuclear translocation and DNA binding in human skin fibroblasts, thus initiating the HS response. No studies have yet been performed on other HSF, and also it is not known whether mild stress activates HSF to the same extent as a severe stress at higher temperatures (Shamovsky and Gershon 2004).

Heat shock proteins (*HSP*): Genes encoding HSP are highly conserved. Many of their products can be assigned to families on the basis of sequence homology and molecular weight. In mammals, many HSP families comprise multiple members that differ in inducibility, intracellular localization and function (Verbeke et al. 2001; Sørensen et al. 2003; Park et al. 2005). HSP are known to play diverse roles as chaperones and/or proteases. In unstressed cells, HSP act in successful folding, assembly, intracellular localization, secretion, regulation and degradation of other proteins. Under conditions in which protein folding is perturbed or proteins begin to unfold and denature, HSP have been shown to assist in protein refolding, to protect cellular systems against protein damages, to dissolve protein aggregates to some extent, to sequester overloaded and damaged proteins into larger aggregates, to target damaged proteins to degradation, and to interfere with the apoptotic programme. Chaperones and proteases can recognise the same protein substrates and the abundance of both types of proteins suggests that HSP are able to distinguish between those proteins that can be refolded and those fated to enter the proteolytic pathway (Söti and Csermely 2000; Söti et al. 2003; Kiang and McClain 2003).

Some HSP are known to be chaperones and are involved in the renaturation of unfolded proteins. Chaperones recognize and bind to other proteins when they are in non-native conformations and are exposing hydrophobic sequences. Their role is to minimize the aggregation of non-native proteins formed during stress. Typically, chaperones function as oligomers, if not as a complex of several different chaperones, co-chaperones and/or nucleotide exchange factors (Feder and Hofmann 1999). In response to heat and oxidative stresses, different small HSP (sHSP) either become phosphorylated or dephosphorylated. Depending on their phosphorylation status, sHSPs form large (300–800 kDa) and active oligomers having an ATP-independent chaperone activity. sHSPs and HSP90 families capture unfolded proteins and create a reservoir of folding intermediates preventing further aggregation. Subsequently, HSP70 and HSP60 families, helped by cochaperones, bind to the stabilized unfolded proteins in the cytosol, mitochondria and endoplasmic reticulum and attempt to restore the structure of proteins in a cycle driven by ATP-hydrolysis. If the target protein is damaged by post-translational modifications, it could be repaired by specific cellular systems before refolding, but such systems exist for only few kinds of damages (Verbeke et al. 2001).

Acting as molecular chaperones, HSP protect many different systems involved in maintenance of cellular functions. sHSP induce an increase of the cellular GSH level leading to the protection of the mitochondrial membrane potential during stress (Préville et al. 1999). HSP70 contains a novel nuclear localisation signal in its C-terminal domain implying a role for HSP70 in the regulation of nuclear proteins and transcription factors such as HSF. Members of HSP70 and HSP90 families are associated with the centrosome, suggesting an involvement in microtubule nucleation or in centrosome assembly. The protection of protein synthesis during stress, called translational thermotolerance, is due to the association of

HSP72 with ribosomal subunits in polysomes of thermotolerant cells. Some chaperones such as the sHSP α_2-crystallin and HSP90 could stabilize a more active conformation of the proteasome (Verbeke et al. 2001).

Members of the HSP90 family constitute 1–2% of cytosolic proteins and have stress-related as well as housekeeping functions. HSP90 stabilize damaged proteins during and after stress. HSP90 interact and either modulate the assembly, the stability and/or the activity of particular cellular proteins such as protein kinases, calcineurin, calmodulin, nitric oxide synthase, telomerase, steroid receptors, oncogenes and transcription factors (Verbeke et al. 2001). HSP90 is presented as a suppressor of cryptic genetic variations by assisting mutant proteins to maintain a wild type structure and function (Rutherford and Lindquist 1998). HSP90 and p23 play also a direct role in the regulation of the HS response by modulating the HSF1 activation/deactivation process. Since HSP90 exists in homeostasis with intracellular hormone receptor and HSF1, it could be hypothesized that steroid hormones activate the HSF by altering this homeostasis. HSP90, HSP70, HSP60 and p23 make heterocomplex with a variety of transcription factors and protein kinases involved in mitogenic signal transduction. The major function of this complex may be to fold the client protein and to keep it inactive until it reaches its ultimate location. There is also a potential involvement of HSP70 and HSP90 in DNA replication since members of these families interact with components of the eukaryotic cell cycle. HSP70, HSP90, HSP27 and TCP-1 are known to bind and stabilize actin, tubulin and the microtubules/microfilament network playing a role in cellular morphology and signal transduction pathways. The HSP60/HSP10 chaperonin system is localized primarily in the matrix space of mitochondria where it assists in folding, refolding and/or elimination of mitochondrial proteins (Kiang and Tsokos 1998; Verbeke et al. 2001).

Our studies show that the basal levels of both the constitutive HSC70 and stress-inducible HSP70 and HSP27 proteins increase during cellular aging of human skin fibroblasts even without any HS (Fonager et al. 2002). A similar increase in the basal level of HSP22 in aged *Drosophila* (King and Tower 1999), and HSP70 in rat kidneys (Maiello et al. 1997) has been reported previously and is taken as the cells' adaptive response to increased intracellular stress during aging. Therefore, it appears that increased levels of HSP27, HSC70 and HSP70 in senescent cells are indicative of their failed attempt to maintain structural and functional ability and to survive for as long as possible. In comparison, exposing these cells to repeated bouts of mild stress stimulates the synthesis of these HSP, maintains their levels high and helps to improve the functional ability and survival of cells without interfering with their replicative lifespan (Fonager et al. 2002). Further analysis of the activities and different modes of action of these HSP and the molecular significance of their increased levels during cellular aging and RMHS treatment is yet to be performed.

In contrast to the increase in the basal level of some HSP discussed above, the basal levels of HSP90 decreased significantly during cellular aging with and without RMHS treatment (Fonager et al. 2002). Although the exact mechanism for the disappearance of HSP90 is not fully understood, it has been proposed that HSP90 during stress binds to partially unfolded proteins and is degraded together with them in a manner similar to what can be observed for HSP70 after HS (Buchner 1999). Furthermore, HSP90 is a powerful modulator of the HS transcription factor HSF1 activation, and the deletion of HSP90 has been shown to promote yeast cells' ability to launch a stress response (Harris et al. 2001). Therefore, it is possible that a decrease in the level of HSP90 during cellular aging and after repeated mild HS treatment is also an adaptive response resulting in the activation of HSF1, which then stimulates the transcription and translation of other HSP.

Some HSP are known to be proteases or to make up the components of a protease system involved in the degradation of the damaged proteins. The irreparable state of a protein could be signalled to the HSP by the extent of irreparable modifications, such as carbonylation (Dukan et al. 2000). HSP70 and its cofactors as well as HSC70, HSP90 are involved in the recognition and the degradation of unnecessary and damaged proteins by the proteasome pathway (*discussed below*). Decreased association of certain proteins with HSP90 and increased association with HSP60/HSP70 lead to their 20S proteasome-mediated degradation. HSP70 has been shown to promote the poly-ubiquitination of damaged proteins. Ubiquitination seems also to be involved in the degradation of unfolded polypeptide by the lysosome. One major mechanism of the lysosomal degradation of proteins is dependent on HSC73 and is responsible for the degradation of a significant amount of the cytosolic protein (Cuervo and Dice 2000).

Protein degradation: One of the main effects of repeated mild HS on human cells is the reduction in the extent of accumulation of oxidatively and glycoxidatively damaged proteins (Verbeke et al. 2000, 2001). Although this may be due to an increase in cellular resistance of RMHS-treated cells to glucose and other protein damaging agents (Verbeke et al. 2002), another possibility is the enhanced removal of abnormal proteins by increased turnover. The bulk of proteolysis is carried out by the ubiquitin-proteasome system in eukaryotes. The proteasome is a multisubunit, multicatalytic proteinase complex, also known as multicatalytic proteinase (MCP). Oxidised proteins are preferentially degraded by the 20S proteasome in an ATP-independent manner, whereas the proteins marked by covalently attached ubiquitin are degraded in an ATP-dependent way by the 26S proteasome, which is ubiquitous among eukaryota, archaebacteria, eubacteria, and prokaryota (Grune 2000; Rivett et al. 2002; Shringaarpure and Davies 2002; Brégégére et al. 2006). The eukaryotic proteasome is present both in the nucleus and in the cytoplasm and constitutes approximately 1% of the total content of cytosolic protein. Polypeptides to be degraded are covalently attached to ubiquitin, which is itself an extremely conserved and heat-inducible HSP. The substrates for the proteasome can be categorised as either misfolded, denatured and otherwise damaged proteins, or perfectly healthy proteins, which have to be removed for normal functioning of the cell, such as cell cycle control, protein quality control, apoptosis and antigen presentation. During aging, there is a decline in the activities of the proteasome, including a decreased activity of the proteasome towards artificial peptide substrates as well as the ability to preferentially degrade oxidized proteins (Brégégére et al. 2006).

We have found that human skin fibroblast cells exposed to repeated mild HS had 20–100% increased proteasome activities, without any accompanied increase in the

20S proteasomal content. However, these hormetic effects of proteasome stimulation by mild heat stress can be dependent on the cell cycle status of the cells. Furthermore, we have observed that this increase in proteasomal activities was related to a significant increase in the amount of the proteasome activator 11S, which is an adaptor between the 20S proteasome and some of the chaperones in the cytosol. The increase of the 20S may be due to an increase in its transcription and translation of 11S activator, an increase in its binding to the 20S proteasome, and a higher level of HSPs in RMHS-treated cells. Although we have not yet determined the extent of transcription, it has been observed that the amount of 11S activartor bound to the 20S proteasome was significantly higher in RMHS-treated cells (Beedholm et al. 2004). Such an increased binding makes it possible for the RMHS-treated cells to activate the proteasome faster than the unstressed cells.

Lysosome is the other major cellular proteolytic system affected by aging. The HSC73-specific lysosomal-proteolytic-pathway is inhibited in senescent fibroblasts (Cuervo and Dice 1996; Cuervo and Dice 2000; Hallén 2002). Accumulation of lipofuscin, which is an aggregate of oxidized proteins and lipids, affects the lysosomal activities (Terman et al. 1999; Terman and Brunk 1998). Other typical cellular inclusions in senescent cells contain over-aggregated proteins as well as chaperones and proteasome components as if both chaperones and proteases have capitulated in face of various insults. A decline in HSF and HSP activity, if not always a decline in their expression, and decrease in the activities of antioxidant enzymes are thought to underlie human neurodegenerative diseases. This is because imbalances of the cellular redox status and lack of chaperone activity promote protein aggregation and favour the development of aging-linked pathologies including cataract, polyglutamine-related disorders or other neurodegenerative diseases as well as cancer (Verbeke et al. 2001; Söti and Csermely 2000; Söti et al. 2003). Severe stress may also promote some of these pathologies more directly by a transcription pathway. Accumulation of oxidized and aggregated proteins could be responsible for the increase in the constitutive expression of some HSPs such as HSP22, HSC70 and HSP70 observed in aged animals, especially in tissues formed by post-mitotic cells exposed to stress for a long period of time (King and Tower 1999). However, no studies have yet been done on the effects of repeated mild HS on lysosome-mediated protein degradation.

Thus, anti-aging hormetic effects of mild HS in aging human cells appear to be facilitated by reducing protein damage and protein aggregation by activating internal antioxidant, repair and degradation processes. HSP are involved in preventing the accumulation of highly damaged proteins during aging since they govern both the repair of weakly damaged proteins and the catabolism of highly damaged proteins. Hormetic pathways are suggested to activate several key proteins involved in the stress response. Indeed, hormesis leads to the maintenance of the HS response during aging and the concomitant transitory and moderate over-expression of HSP in cells and organisms is greatly beneficial. However, the extent of the beneficial effects of HS are also affected by the genotype, as shown by the observed differences in HS response of human lymphocytes in the context of polymorphism in HSP70 genes (Singh et al. 2004; Singh et al. 2006; Singh et al. 2006; Singh et al. 2007).

Cold shock: Almost all the studies described above have used HS at temperatures higher than the normal body temperature. There are no systematic and long-term studies performed on the effects of single or multiple exposures of normal human cells to lower temperatures. In Chinese hamster ovary cells, hypothermia-induced cold stress is reported to increase their resistance to hydrogen peroxide-induced apoptosis by enhancing the expression of bcl-2 gene (Slikker et al. 2001). Similarly, in the case of isolated mesenchymal stem cells from young and old rats, exposure to hypothermia at 32 °C increased the levels of some stress proteins, and reduced the levels of reactive oxygen species (ROS) and carbonylated abnormal proteins (Stolzing et al. 2006). It will be interesting to elucidate the effects of mild and severe cold shock on age-related changes in human cells, which will be useful in making a distinction between general stress response and temperature-specific stress response, and its applicability as hormetic agents.

Other Hormetic Stress Treatments in Aging Human Cells

Irradiation, mechanical stress, cortisols, proxidants and some natural and synthetic molecules are some of the other potential hormetic agents tested for their beneficial and anti-aging effects on human cells. For example, a very low dose rate of chronic ionizing radiation increased the division potential of human embryonic lung fibroblasts WI-38 (Icard et al. 1979; Croute et al. 1986). Similarly, the adaptive response of human embryonic cells to low dose gamma-radiation has been shown to increase the replicative lifespan by up to 160% compared to non-irradiated cells (Watanabe et al. 1992). Furthermore, human embryonic lung fibroblasts MRC-5 sequentially irradiated with 1 Gy gamma rays had their replicative lifespan increased to some extent (Holliday 1991). Hormetic effects of low dose X-irradiation on the proliferative ability, genomic stability and activation of mitogen-activated protein kinase pathways have been reported for other human diploid cells including embryonic fibroblasts (Tsutsui et al. 1997; Suzuki et al. 1998; Suzuki et al. 2001; Suzuki et al. 1998; Yang et al. 1998). Similarly, repetitive low-dose UVA irradiation of human skin fibroblasts enhanced their antioxidative ability and increased resistance to phototoxicity under selenium deficient conditions (Meewes et al. 2001). Recent studies on the exposure of human skin fibroblasts and keratinocytes to 900 MHz (GSM-900) radiofrequency radiation for 48 h showed an induction of HSP70, which can have some protective effects in terms of its chaperoning activity (Sanchez et al. 2006).

Other mild stress treatments which have been shown to have some beneficial hormetic effects in human cells include glucocorticoids in skin fibroblasts from Cushing's syndrome patients (Pratsinis et al. 2002; Zervolea et al. 2005), hydrogen peroxide in umbilical vein endothelial cells (HUVEC) and keratinocytes (Haendeler et al. 2004; Yokoo et al. 2004), and nitric oxide (NO) in keratinocytes (Krischel et al. 1998). Shear stressing of HUVEC in parallel plate flow chamber induced changes in gene expression including enhanced NO production and cytochrome

P450 expression (McCormick et al. 2001). However, no long-term studies on determining the effects of shear stress on age-related changes in human cells have yet been performed. With respect to nutritional stress, our preliminary studies have shown that partial food restriction by serum starvation (2% serum instead of normal 10% serum) of human skin fibroblasts for 24 h once a week increases their lysosomal autophagic activity, reduces the accumulation of intracellular debris, and enhances the replicative lifespan (*unpublished observations*).

Some natural and synthetic molecules which appear to have anti-aging effects on human cells through stress-induced maintenance and repair are also being tested, and these are collectively termed as hormetins (Ali and Rattan 2006; Rattan and Ali 2007). Such potential hormetins include thymidine dimers which enhance DNA repair in human keratinocytes (Eller et al. 1997) and enhance melanin production in melanocytes (Lin and Fisher 2007), celastrols from certain Chinese herbs which induce HS response (Westerheide et al. 2004), and curcumin which stimulates proteasome activity, sodium pump activity and HS response in human keratinocytes (Ali and Rattan 2006; Rattan and Ali 2007). It will be useful to test other natural and synteitc compounds which may be potential hormetins for human cells in culture and for other experimental model systems of aging.

Conclusions

The Hayflick system of cellular aging *in vitro* has facilitated testing the hormesis hypothesis of anti-aging modulation in human cells. That repeated mild stress, followed by a period of recovery and adaptation, has a wide range of biological effects which are generally beneficial is now well documented in this experimental system. At the cellular and molecular level it has been shown that the major pathways of hormetic response include heat shock proteins, other chaperones, antioxidant defenses, proteasomal and lysosomal activities and DNA repair systems. Studies performed on human cells in culture have provided the proof of the principle that hormetic modulation of the process of aging is a real possibility. The results obtained from cell culture studies can also be the basis for elucidating the mechanisms of hormetic effects of other stresses such as exercise, calorie restriction, nutritional components, and psychosocial factors.

References

Ali RE, Rattan SIS (2006) Curcumin's biphasic hormetic response on proteasome activity and heat shock protein synthesis in human keratinocytes. Ann NY Acad Sci 1067: 394–399

Beedholm R, Clark BFC, Rattan SIS (2004) Mild heat stress stimulates proteasome and its 11S activator in human fibroblasts undergoing aging in vitro. Cell Stress Chaperones 9: 49–57

Berge U, Behrens J, Rattan SIS (2007) Sugar-induced premature aging and altered differentiation in human epidermal keratinocytes. Ann NY Acad Sci 1100: 524–529

Brégégére F, Milner Y, Friguet B (2006) The ubiquitin-proteasome system at the crossroads of stress-response and ageing pathways: a handle for skin care? Aging Res Rev 5: 60–90
Buchner J (1999) Hsp90 & co. – a holding for folding. TIBS 24: 136–141
Croute F, Vidal S, Soleilhavoup JP, Vincent C, Serre G, Planel H (1986) Effects of a very low dose rate of chronic ionizing radiation on the division potential of human embryonic lung fibroblasts in vitro. Exp Gerontol 21: 1–11
Cuervo AM, Dice JF (1996) A receptor for the selective uptake and degradation of proteins by lysosomes. Science 273: 501–503
Cuervo AM, Dice JF (2000) When lysosomes get old. Exp Gerontol 35: 119–131
Dorion S, Landry J (2002) Activation of the mitogen-activated protein kinase pathways by heat shock. Cell Stress Chaperones 7: 200–206
Dukan S, Farewell A, Ballesteros M, Taddei F, Rodman M, Nyström T (2000) Protein oxidation in response to increased transcriptional or translational errors. Proc Natl Acad Sci USA 97: 5746–5749
Eller MS, Maeda T, Magnoni C, Atwal D, Gilchrest BA (1997) Enhancement of DNA repair in human skin cells by thymidine dinucleotides: evidence for a p53-mediated mammalian SOS response. Proc Natl Acad Sci USA 94: 12627–12632
Feder ME, Hofmann GE (1999) Heat-shock proteins, molecular chaperones, and the stress response. Annu Rev Physiol 61: 243–282
Fonager J, Beedholm R, Clark BFC, Rattan SIS (2002) Mild stress-induced stimulation of heat shock protein synthesis and improved functional ability of human fibroblasts undergoing aging in vitro. Exp Gerontol 37: 1223–1238
Gabai VL, Meriin AB, Yaglom JA, Volloch VZ, Sherman MY (1998) Role of Hsp70 in regulation of stress-kinase JNK: implications in apoptosis and aging. FEBS Lett 438: 1–4.
Gabai VL, Sherman MY (2002) Interplay between molecular chaperones and signaling pathways in survival of heat shock. J Appl Physiol 92: 1743–1748
Grune T (2000) Oxidative stress, aging and the proteasomal system. Biogerontology 1: 31–40.
Haendeler J, Tischler V, Hoffmann J, Zeiher AM, Dimmeler S (2004) Low doses of reactive oxygen species protects endothelial cells from apoptosis byincreasing thioredo. FEBS Lett 577: 427–433
Hallén A (2002) Accumulation of insoluble protein and aging. Biogerontology 3: 307–315.
Harris N, MacLean M, Hatzianthis K, Panaretou B, Piper PW (2001) Increasing Saccharomyces cerevisiae stress resistance, through the overactivation of the heat shock response resulting from defects in the Hsp90 chaperone, does not extend replicative life span but can be associated with slower chronological ageing of nondividing cells. Mol Genet Genomics 265: 258–263
Holliday R (1991) A re-examination of the effects of ionizing radiation on lifespan and transformation of human diploid fibroblasts. Mutat Res 256: 295–302
Icard C, Beupain R, Dialtoff C, Macieira-Coelho A (1979) Effect of low dose rate irradiation on the division potential of cells in vitro. VI. changes in DNA and in radiosensitivity during aging of human fibroblasts. Mech Age Develop 11: 269–278
Kaul SC, Wadhwa R, Eds. (2003) Aging of cells in and outside the body. Dordrecht, Kluwer
Kiang JG, McClain DE (2003) Heat stress. In: Tsokos, GC, Atkins, JL (Eds). Combat Medicine: Basic and Clinical Research in Military, Trauma, and Emergency Medicine, pp. 83–101, NJ, Humana
Kiang JG, McClain DE, Warke VG, Krishnan S, Tsokos GC (2003) Constitutive NO synthase regulates the Na+/Ca2+ exchanger in human T cells: role of [Ca2+]i and tyrosine phosphorylation. J Cell Biochem 89: 1030–1043
Kiang JG, Tsokos GC (1998) Heat shock protein 70kDa: molecular biology, biochemistry, and physiology. Pharmacol Ther 80: 183–201
King V, Tower, J (1999) Aging-specific expression of *Drosophila hsp22*. Dev Biol 207: 107–118
Kraft DC, Deocaris CC, Rattan SIS (2006) Proteasomal oscillation during mild heat shock in aging human skin fibroblasts. Ann NY Acad Sci 1067: 224–227

Krischel V, Bruch-Gerharz D, Suschek C, Kröncke KD, Ruzicka T, Kolb-Bachofen V (1998) Biphasic effects of exogenous nitric oxide on proliferation and differentation in skin derived keratinocytes but not fibroblasts. J Invest Dermatol 111: 286–291
Lin JY, Fisher DE (2007) Melanocyte biology and skin pigmentation. Nature 445: 843–850
Maiello M, Boeri D, Sampietro L, Pronzato MA, Odetti P, Marinari UM (1997) Basal synthesis of heat shock protein 70 increases with age in rat kidneys. Gerontology 44: 15–20
McCormick SM, Eskin SG, McIntire LV, Teng CL, Lu CM, Russell CG, Chittur KK (2001) DNA microarray reveals changes in gene expression of shear stressed human umbilical vein endothelial cells. Proc Natl Acad Sci USA 98: 8955–8960
Meewes C, Brenneisen P, Wenk J, Kuhr L, Ma W, Alikoski J, Poswig A, Kreig T, et al. (2001) Adaptive antioxidant response protects dermal fibroblasts from UVA-induced phototoxicity. Free Rad Biol Med 30: 238–247
Meriin AB, Yaglom JA, Gabai VL, Zon L, Ganiatsas S, Mosser DD, Sherman MY (1999) Protein-damaging stresses activate c-Jun N-terminal kinase via inhibition of its dephosphorylation: a novel pathway controlled by HSP72. Mol Cell Biol 19: 2547–2555
Nielsen ER, Eskildsen-Helmond Y, Rattan SIS (2006) MAP-kinases and heat shock-induced hormesis in human fibroblasts during serial passaging in vitro. Ann NY Acad Sci 1067: 343–348
Nørgaard R, Kassem M, Rattan SIS (2006) Heat shock-induced enhancement of osteoblastic differentiation of hTERT-immortlized mesenchymal stem cells. Ann NY Acad Sci 1067: 443–447
Park HG, Han SI, Oh SY, Kang HS (2005) Cellular responses to mild heat stress. Cell Mol Life Sci 62: 10–23
Park J, Liu YC (2001) JNK phosphorylates the HSF1 transcriptional activation domain: role of JNK in the regulation of the heat shock response. J Cell Biochem 82: 326–338
Pratsinis H, Tsagarakis S, Zervolea I, Giannakopoulos F, Stathakos D, Thalassinos N, Kletsas D (2002) Chronic in vivo exposure to glucocorticoids prolongs cellular lifespan: the case of Cushing's syndrome-patients' fibroblasts. Exp Gerontol 37: 1237–1245
Préville X, Salvemini F, Giraud S, Chafour S, Paul C, Stepien G, Ursini MV, Arrigo AP (1999) Mammalian small stress proteins protect against oxidative stress through their ability to increase glucose-6-phosphate dehydrogenease activity and by maintaining optimal cellular detoxifying machinery. Exp Cell Res 247: 61–78
Rattan SIS (2001) Applying hormesis in aging research and therapy. Hum Exp Toxicol 20: 281–285
Rattan SIS (1998) Repeated mild heat shock delays ageing in cultured human skin fibroblasts. Biochem Mol Biol Int 45: 753–759
Rattan SIS (2003) Aging outside the body: usefulness of the Hayflick system. In: Kaul, SC, Wadhwa, R (Eds). Aging of Cells In and Outside the Body, pp. 1–8, Dordrecht, Kluwer
Rattan SIS (2004) Aging intervention, prevention, and therapy through hormesis. J Gerontol Biol Sci 59A: 705–709
Rattan SIS (2006) Theories of biological aging: genes, proteins and free radicals. Free Rad Res 40: 1230–1238
Rattan SIS, Ali, RE (2007) Hormetic prevention of molecular damage during cellular aging of human fibroblasts and keratinocytes. Ann NY Acad Sci 1100: 424–430
Rivett AJ, Bose S, Pemberton AJ, Brooks P, Onion D, Shirley D, Stratford FLL, Forti K (2002) Assay of proteasome activity in relation to aging. Exp Gerontol 37: 1217–1222
Rutherford SL, Lindquist S (1998) Hsp90 as a capacitor for morphological evolution. Nature 396: 336–342
Salvioli S, Bonafe M, Capri M, Monti D, Franceschi C (2001) Mitochondria, aging and longevity – a new perspective. FEBS Lett 492: 9–13
Sanchez S, Milochau A, Ruffie G, de Gannes FP, Lagroye, I, Haro E, Surleve-Bazeille JE, Billaudel B, et al. (2006) Human skin cell stress response to GSM-900 mobile phone signals. In vitro study on isolated primary cells and reconstructed epidermis. FEBS J 273: 5491–5507

Shamovsky I, Gershon D (2004) Novel regulatory factors of HSF-1 activation: facts and perspectives regarding their involevement in the age-associated attenauation of the heat shock response. Mech Age Dev 125: 767–775

Shringaarpure R, Davies KJA (2002) Protein turnover by the proteasome in aging and disease. Free Rad Biol Med 32: 1084–1089

Singh R, Kølvraa S, Bross P, Christensen K, Gregersen N, Tan Q, Jensen UB, Eiberg H, et al. (2006) Heat-shock protein 70 genes and human longevity. A view from Denmark. Ann NY Acad Sci 1067: 301–308

Singh R, Kølvraa S, Bross P, Gregersen N, Nexø BA, Frederiksen H, Christensen K, Rattan SIS (2004) Association between low self-rated health and heterozygosity for −110A-C polymorphism in the promoter region of HSP70–1 in aged Danish twins. Biogerontology 5: 169–176

Singh R, Kølvraa S, Bross P, Jensen UB, Gregersen N, Tan Q, Knudese C, Rattan SIS (2006) Reduced heat shock response in human mononuclear cells during aging and its association with polymorphisms on HSP70 genes. Cell Stress Chaperones 11: 208–215

Singh R, Kølvraa S, Rattan SIS (2007) Genetics of longevity with emphasis on the relevance of HSP70 genes. Frontiers in Biology 12: 4504–4513

Slikker W, Desai VG, Duhart H, Feuers R, Imam SZ (2001) Hypothermia enhances bcl-2 expression and protects against oxidative stress-induced cell death in Chinese hamster ovary cells. Free Rad Biol Med 31: 405–411

Söti C, Csermely P (2000) Molecular chaperones and the aging process. Biogerontology 1: 225–233

Söti C, Pál C, Papp B, Csermely P (2005) Molecular chaperones as regulatory elements of cellular networks. Curr Opin Cell Biol 17: 210–215

Söti C, Sreedhar AS, Csermely P (2003) Apoptosis, necrosis and cellular senescence: chaperone occupancy as a potential switch. Aging Cell 2: 39–45

Sørensen JG, Kristensen TN, Loeschcke V (2003) The evolutionary and ecological role of heat shock proteins. Ecol Lett 6: 1025–1037

Stolzing A, Sethe S, Scutt A (2006) Stressed stem cells: temperature response in aged mesenchymal stem cells. Stem Cells and Dev 15: 478–487

Sun Y, MacRae TH (2005) The small heat shock proteins and their role in human disease. FEBS J 272: 2613–2627

Suzuki K, Kodama S, Watanabe M (1998) Suppressive effects of low-dose preirradiation on genetic instability induced by X rays in normal embryonic cells. Radiat Res 150: 656–662.

Suzuki K, Kodama S, Watanabe M (2001) Extremely low-dose ionizing radiation causes activation of mitogen-activated protein kinase pathway and enhances proliferation of normal human diploid cells. Cancer Res 61: 5396–5401

Suzuki M, Yang Z, Nakano K, Yatagai F, Suzuki K, Kodama S, Watanabe M (1998) Extension of in vitro life-span of gamma-irradiated human embryo cells accompanied by chromosome instability. J Radiat Res 39: 203–213

Terman A, Abrahamsson N, Brunk UT (1999) Ceroid/lipofuscin-loaded human fibroblasts show increased susceptibility to oxidative stress. Exp Gerontol 34: 755–770

Terman A, Brunk UT (1998) Ceroid/lipofuscin formation in cultured human fibroblasts: the role of oxidative stress and proteolysis. Mech Age Dev. 104: 277–291

Tsutsui T, Tanaka Y, Matsudo Y, Hasegawa K, Fujino T, Kodama S, Barrett JC (1997) Extended lifespan and immortalization of human fibroblasts induced by X-ray irradiation. Mol Carcinog 18: 7–18

Verbeke P, Clark BFC, Rattan SIS (2000) Modulating cellular aging in vitro: hormetic effects of repeated mild heat stress on protein oxidation and glycation. Exp Gerontol 35: 787–794

Verbeke P, Clark BFC, Rattan SIS (2001) Reduced levels of oxidized and glycoxidized proteins in human fibroblasts exposed to repeated mild heat shock during serial passaging in vitro. Free Rad Biol Med 31: 1593–1602

Verbeke P, Deries M, Clark BFC, Rattan SIS (2002) Hormetic action of mild heat stress decreases the inducibility of protein oxidation and glycoxidation in human fibroblasts. Biogerontology 3: 105–108

Verbeke P, Fonager J, Clark BFC, Rattan SIS (2001) Heat shock response and ageing: mechanisms and applications. Cell Biol Int 25: 845–857

Watanabe M, Suzuki M, Suzuki K, Nakano K, Watanabe K (1992) Effect of multiple irradiation with low doses of gamma-rays on morphological transformation and growth ability of human embryo cells in vitro. Int J Radiat Biol 62: 711–718

Westerheide SD, Bosman JD, Mbadugha BNA, Kawahara TLA, Matsumoto G, Kim S, Gu W, Devlin JP, et al. (2004) Celastrols as inducers of the heat shock response and cytoprotection. J Biol Chem 279: 56053–56060

Yang Z, Kodama S, Suzuki K, Watanabe K (1998) Telomerase activity, telomere length, and chromosome aberrations in the extension of life span of human embryo cells induced by low-lose X-rays. J Radiat Res 39: 35–51

Yokoo S, Furumoto K, Hiyama E, Miwa N (2004) Slow down of age-dependent telomere shortening is executed in human skin keratinocytes by hormesis-like-effects of trace hydrogen peroxide or by antioxidative effects of pro-vitamin C in common concurrently with reduction of intracellular oxidative stress. J Cell Biochem 93: 588–597

Zervolea I, Pratsinis H, Tsagarakis S, Karavitaki N, Stathakos D, Thalassinos N, Kletsas D (2005) The impact of chronic in vivo glucocorticoid excess on the functional characteristics of human skin fibroblasts obtained from patients with endogeneous Cushing's syndrome. Eur J Endocrinol 152: 895–902

Chapter 7
Physical Activity: A Strong Stimulant for Hormesis During Aging

Li Li Ji[1]

Introduction: Physical Activity and Successful Aging

In the animal world physical exercise is an intimate part of life cycle to pursue food, escape predators, and ensure reproduction. Aged individuals with reduced fitness and mobility are subjected to natural selection. In rodents, volunteer wheel runners show an increase in both maximal life span and 50% survival rate compared to their sedentary counterparts, indicating physical activity can change aging process (Holloszy 1993). In human population, morbidity is concentrated in the last 2 decades of life, beginning on the average at age 55 and increasing in frequency until the average age of death at 75. The benefit of exercise is highlighted by the increase of approximately 2 years in longevity in physically active people as compared to less active people (Paffenbarger et al. 1993). Disability levels in a vigorously exercising population are below that of non-exercisers and age-related increases in disability are delayed by approximately 15 years (Fries 1996). These data indicate that engaging in regular physical activity would increase the age of onset of chronic illness and shorten the time between the onset of morbidity and death. Furthermore, this compression of the period of morbidity as a result of physical exercise would represent a significant improvement in the quality of life and result in major reductions in the health care for the elderly.

Despite these clear benefits of participating in physical exercise, there is a concern that aged individuals are more susceptible to some of the harmful effects of rigorous exercise as a result of increased exposure to reactive oxygen species (ROS) (Davies et al. 1982). The free radical theory of aging (Harman 1956) has allowed for the establishment of a powerful link between exercise and aging research. A fundamental premise for this theory is that ROS generated in normal metabolic processes are the underlying reason for cell and tissue oxidative damage seen throughout the aging process. Since exercise increases metabolic rate reflected by

[1]The Biodynamics Laboratory, Department of Kinesiology, University of Wisconsin-Madison, Madison, WI 53706, USA.

Address for correspondence:
2000 Observatory Drive, Madison, WI 53706, USA. Tel: (608) 262-7250; Fax: (608) 262-1656; e-mail: ji@education.wisc.edu

E. Le Bourg and S.I.S. Rattan (eds.), *Mild Stress and Healthy Aging.*

a greater amount of oxygen uptake, ROS production is increased during physical exertion. One may naturally ask this question: is physical exercise more beneficial or harmful to the elderly population? A complete and unequivocal conclusion is still forthcoming; however, there is enough evidence to demonstrate that a mild oxidative stress associate with exercise may not be a bad thing during aging.

Although aging may cause increased ROS generation and oxidative stress probably in all cell types, which could be influenced by physical activity overall, in this chapter the author chose to focus on skeletal muscle for the obvious reasons that (a) skeletal muscle health is vital for mobility and normal life; (b) deterioration of skeletal muscle mass and functionality (sarcopenia) is an important issue in medical gerontology (Thomas 2007); and (c) skeletal muscle has displayed some unique characteristics during aging.

Exercise and Oxidative Stress

The most prominent biological changes occurring during exercise is the increased metabolic rate, matched by an enhanced rate of mitochondrial respiration and oxidative phosphorylation to provide ATP for contracting muscles. It is estimated that during maximal workload in men oxygen consumption at the local muscle fibers can reach as high as 100-fold of the resting levels, while the whole body oxygen consumption (VO_2) increases by ~20-fold. The electron transport chain (ETC) consumes >85% of all the O_2 utilized in the cell whereas ~1–5% of oxygen can form $O_2^{\bullet-}$ and eventually other ROS as byproducts (Meydani and Evans 1993). A large number of studies reported elevated $O_2^{\bullet-}$ level in skeletal muscle following contractile activity (see Ji 1999). For example, using dichlorofluorescin (DCFH), a non-specific intracellular ROS probe Bejma and Ji (1999) showed that an acute bout of treadmill running at 75% VO_2 max for 1 h can increase ROS production by 30–40%, corresponding to 20–30 pmol/min/mg protein in rat quadriceps muscles. Using a microdialysis technique, McArdle et al. (2001) reported a mean amount of 1.2 nmol $O_2^{\bullet-}$ in contracting mouse gastrocnemius muscle during the 15 min period of electrically stimulated contraction. It is important to point out that the observed elevation of ROS was in spite of the continuous removal by endogenous antioxidant defense systems, composed of superoxide dismutase (SOD), catalase (CAT) and glutathione peroxidase (GPX), as well as ROS scavengers such as vitamin E, C and GSH.

Mitochondria are the main, but not the only source of ROS during muscle contraction. Depending on the intensity of exercise and the physiological conditions, several other cellular components and pathways can contribute to ROS production. Xanthine oxidase (XO) plays a major role in $O_2^{\bullet-}$ production in skeletal muscle during intermittent hypoxia and reoxygenation, which occurs during ischemic contraction, heavy weight lifting and sprinting exercise (Gomez-Cabrera et al. 2005). Member-borne NADPH oxidase can be activated to generate $O_2^{\bullet-}$ during muscle contraction (Bejma and Ji 1999; Pattwell et al. 2004) and injury-associated inflammation (see below).

Another important source of ROS during muscle contraction is nitric oxide (NO) (Reid 2001). Several authors demonstrated increased NO production in cultured myotubes in vitro (Pattwell et al. 2004), in isolated contracting muscle (Balon 1999), and in muscle subjected to passive stretching (Tidball et al. 1998). The major enzyme producing NO in muscle cells are endothelial NO synthase (eNOS); however, inducible NOS (iNOS) may increase its importance when muscle undergoes lengthening contraction (LC), inflammation and healing (Sakurai et al. 2005). While the increased NO can scavenge $O_2^{\bullet-}$ to reduce $^{\bullet}OH$ formation via Haber-Weise reaction, it risks the generation of peroxynitrite, another highly reactive species that targets selective amino acids such as phenoalanine and tyrosine (Leeuwenburgh et al. 1999).

Physical activity at high intensity sometimes leads to mechanical injury such as stretching or muscle-soft tissue injury followed by inflammation. Inflammatory cells in the injured tissues can generate ROS (Cannon and Blumberg 1994). Blood-borne polymorphoneutrophils (PMN) play a critical role in defending tissues from viral and bacterial infection by producing $O_2^{\bullet-}$ via activation of NADPH oxidase during a respiratory burst (Pyne 1994; Aoi et al. 2004). Cytoplasmic (CuZn) SOD converts $O_2^{\bullet-}$ to H_2O_2, which is further converted to $^{\bullet}OH$ in the presence of ferrous ions, or to hydrochloric acid (HOCl) catalyzed by myleoperoxidase. While these ROS are considered critical in the healing process, they can also cause secondary damage to healthy muscle cells. Figure 1 illustrates major cellular sources of ROS during exercise or inflammation.

Aging Increases Exercise-Induced Oxidative Stress

Aging increases ROS production in the cell especially in the mitochondria (Sohal and Sohal 1991). In skeletal muscle and heart ROS production is also increased with age along with increased oxidative damage markers. ROS production was shown to be 77% higher in the muscle of 25 month-old rats than 8 month-old rats, and increased 50% and 38%, respectively after 1 h treadmill running (Bejma and Ji 1999). In the above study running speed and grade were adjusted to impose a similar workload (~75% VO_2max) to the young and old rats. In the heart, ROS production was also increased with age, but the acute exercise bout increased ROS generation only in the old rat (Bejma et al. 2000). These data clearly reveal that as animals grow older, a smaller work task can provoke a greater ROS-generating effect in the heart and skeletal muscle.

The reason for the aged animals to increase ROS production during exercise is not entirely clear. Age-related defects in mitochondrial ETC are considered a major mechanism (Nolh et al. 1978; McArdle and Jackson 2000). Lowered cytochrome c oxidase (complex IV) with age favors a greater electron "leakage" and formation of $O_2^{\bullet-}$ in the senescent organism. Peroxidative modification of mitochondrial membrane lipids may be another major change at old age, such as elevated malondialdehyde and 4-hydroxynonenol levels, decreased membrane fluidity and enhanced fatty acid unsaturation (Kim et al. 1996; Yu and Chung 2006). These changes may

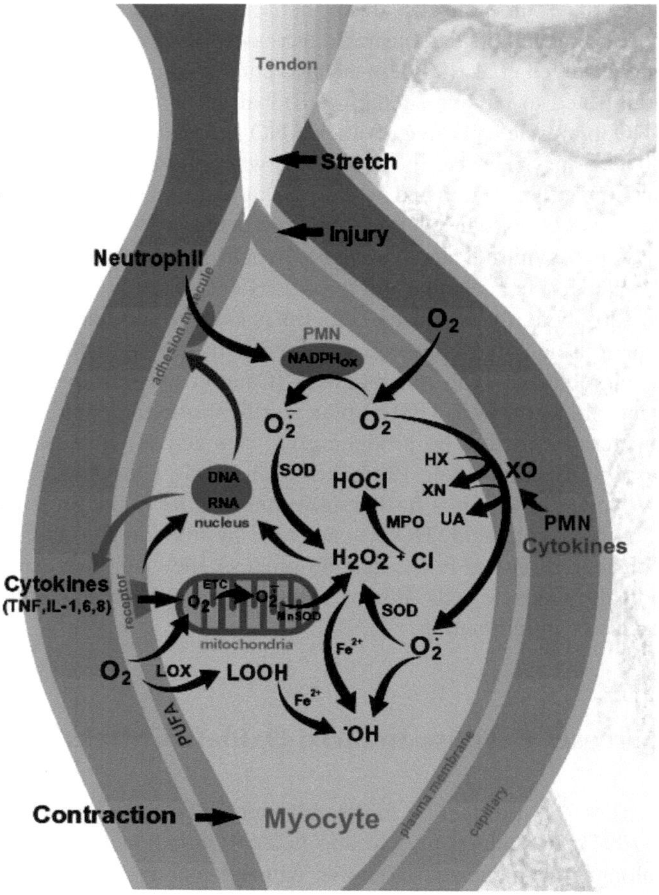

Fig. 1 Sources of reactive oxygen species (ROS) in muscle cells during exercise and contraction-mediated injury. Abbreviations: ETC, election transport chain; HOCl, hypochorous acid; HX, hypoxanthine; IL, interleukine; LOX, lipooxygenase; MPO, melyeoperoxidase; PMN, polymorphoneutrophil; SOD, superoxide dismutase; TNF-α, tumor necrosis factor-α; UA, uric acid; XN, xanthine; XO, xanthine oxidase

cause further ROS generation via ETC and enzymatic pathways involving cyclooxygenase (COX), NADPH oxidase and XO (Sawada et al. 1992).

Chronic muscle inflammation is a common problem associated with old age. Endothelial cells from injured muscle are known to release cytokines such as tumor necrosis factor (TNF)-α, interleukin (IL)-1 and 6 with distinct individual time courses (Pedersen et al. 1998). These pro-inflammatory molecules can stimulate signal transduction pathways (see below) to promote de novo expression of the above cytokines and vascular cellular adhesion molecules (VCAM). Increased iNOS expression and subsequent NO production may cause vasodilation that further facilitates PMN and cytokine infiltration, forming a vicious cycle (Gath et al. 1996). All these events may occur several hours to a few days after an acute bout of strenuous exercise, especially when involving LC (Best et al. 1999). Aged individuals are more susceptible to muscle injury as a much smaller workload can produce mechanical injury. In humans, stretch injury and fall constitute a majority of incidence for subsequent muscle inflammation.

Antioxidant Defense in Aging Muscle: A Hormetic Response?

Aging is associated with a deterioration of protein synthesis and cell differentiation capacity in most tissues, particularly in the postmitotic tissues. Therefore, antioxidant utilization and degradation probably are not adequately replenished at old age. However, antioxidants have demonstrated considerable plasticity in response to oxidant exposure. Localized oxidative stress in specific organelles and cell compartments may stimulate cellular uptake and synthesis of certain antioxidants under highly regulated signaling process (Ji 2007). According to the free radical theory of aging one might expect to see a general decline of cellular antioxidant defense capacity at old age. Available data suggest that these changes are not uniform across all species and all cell types, and some even show an increased antioxidant defense with age (Matsuo 1993). Skeletal muscle is a unique organ that exhibits marked increases in antioxidant enzyme activity with aging (Ji et al. 1990; Lawler et al. 1993; Luhtala et al. 1994). Activities of all major antioxidant enzymes, such as SOD, CAT and GPX, as well as GSH sulfur-transferase and glutathione reductase, were significantly higher in the hindlimb muscles of old vs. young rats. In order to know whether gene expression of antioxidant enzymes are more active in skeletal muscle of age animals, mRNA levels and enzyme protein contents were measured for the various enzymes. All studies did not find significant changes of the relative abundance of mRNA for either SOD isozyme or GPX, except for CAT mRNA which showed an increase with age in soleus muscle (see Ji 2001). Age-adaptation of antioxidant enzymes appears to be muscle fiber specific, with the most prominent increases found in type 1 (slow-twitch oxidative) muscles, followed by type 2a (fast-twitch oxidative), whereas type 2b muscles showed little effect. Luhtala et al. (1994) reported that elevation of muscle antioxidant enzymes during aging was markedly affected by dietary restriction in Fischer 344 rats. The progressive increases in CAT and GPX activities from 11 to 34 month of age were prevented by a 30% reduction of food intake, while an age-related increase in MnSOD was also attenuated.

Aging is associated with a decline of cellular thiol reserve in most tissues (Matsuo 1993). However, skeletal muscle and heart may be spared of this effect. Leeuwenburgh et al. (1994) showed that aging caused no significant alteration of GSH content or GSH/GSSG ratio in rat deep vastus lateralis (DVL) muscle, whereas in soleus there was a 37% increase in GSH content in old rats along with a higher GSH/GSSG ratio. Activity of γ-glutamyl transpeptidase (GGT), the first enzyme in the γ-glutamyl cycle, was elevated in the aged muscle indicative of a greater potential for muscle GSH transport. Fiebig et al. (1996) showed a significant increase in total glutathione content (GSH + GSSG) in the heart of 27- vs. 5-month-old rats. The elevated myocardial GSH content was associated with a twofold increase in GGT activity.

The mechanism responsible for the increased antioxidant enzyme activities in aging skeletal muscle is still elusive. Mitochondria from aged muscles produce more ROS that may stimulate antioxidant enzyme gene expression. This scenario is consistent with the finding that mitochondrial fractions of antioxidant enzyme activity showed a greater increase in the senescent skeletal muscle (Ji et al. 1990; Luhtala et al. 1994). Age-related muscle inflammation and ROS production through NADPH oxidase and NOS may also play a role (Yu and Chung 2006). The lack of uniformity in mRNA elevation of antioxidant enzymes suggests that age-related adaptation is complicated and subject to both transcriptional and post-transcriptional mechanisms yet to be understood. Recent findings of age-related alteration in cell signaling may shed some light on this issue (see below).

Muscle Contraction: A Powerful Stimulant for Antioxidant Adaptation

Although aged muscles demonstrated higher levels of ROS generation when they were subjected to an acute bout of exercise at a given workload, animals or humans involved in chronic exercise training demonstrate lower levels of oxidative stress and damage at the organ, tissue and cell levels as documented by numerous research (Sen 1995; Meydani and Evans 1993; Powers et al. 1999). For example, "trained" muscles have shown lower levels of lipid peroxidation, protein oxidation, DNA damage and disturbance of redox status both at rest and in response to an acute bout of exercise. Muscle mitochondria isolated from trained rats showed greater resistance to imposed oxidants and improved respiratory function (Chandwaney et al. 1998; Tonkonogi and Sahlin 2002). Hearts of animals involved in endurance training are less susceptible to ischemia-reperfusion insult either in vitro (i.e., isolated perfused model), in situ (e.g., open heart surgery model) or in vivo (Bowles et al. 1992; Ramires and Ji 2001). The benefits of chronic exercise are not limited to skeletal muscle and heart. Liver, brain, erythrocytes and other tissues from animals or humans engaged in routine exercise demonstrate a lesser extent of oxidative damage as compared to their sedentary counterparts (Goto et al. 2007). Interestingly, these changes are associated with increased muscle and whole body oxygen consumption, increased utilization of fat as energy fuel, and increase muscle mitochondrial population, which all seem to favor a higher level of ROS generation.

Numerous studies have shown that antioxidant enzyme activities are elevated in skeletal muscle after endurance training involving repeated bouts of prolonged exercise, and this is probably the most important reason as to why training reduces oxidative stress in young as well as old individuals. Due to the abundance of reviews on this subject (see Power et al. 1999; Ji 1999, 2007; Reid 2001; Jackson 2005), only a brief summary of the findings is provided below. (a) Among antioxidant enzymes in skeletal muscle, SOD activity has consistently been shown to increase with exercise training in an intensity-dependent manner. MnSOD is primarily responsible for the observed increase in SOD activity, whereas CuZn SOD activity is little affected. GPX activity has also shown an increase after endurance training by most authors. Training effect on CAT activity is inconsistent and controversial. Muscle fiber type is an important factor in determining whether and how much training can influence antioxidant enzyme activity, reflecting both fiber recruitment patterns during exercise and intrinsic antioxidant capacity within a given fiber. Myocardial and diaphragm SOD and GPX have also been shown to increase with treadmill running and swim training in rats. (b) There is considerable evidence that the observed training adaptation of antioxidant activity is due to altered gene expression, with both mRNA and enzyme protein levels being upregulated. For example, resting MnSOD activity and protein content were increased with endurance training in several rat muscles. Even though resting mRNA level for MnSOD was not affected by training status, it was elevated immediately following an acute bout of exercise. Since mRNA generally has a short half-life and muscle tissues in the above studies were harvested 24–48 h post-exercise, it can be concluded that mRNA may increase only transiently following acute exercise bouts. In contrast to SOD, available data indicate that steady state GPX and CAT mRNA levels in trained rat muscles are not different from the sedentary controls, whereas their acute response to exercise is little known.

Training can elicit whole-body adaptations that benefit individual organs and tissues to battle against deleterious ROS. This notion could be supported by two important systems, i.e., GSH and cytokines modulation. GSH is a required antioxidant for all cells, whereas de novo synthesis of GSH occurs only in the liver. Thus, most organs including skeletal muscle and heart import GSH from the circulation via the γ-glutamyl cycle (Meister and Anderson 1983). Exercise training has been shown to induce hepatic γ-glutamylcysteinyl synthetase (GCS), the rate-limiting enzyme for GSH synthesis (Ramires and Ji 2001). GGT activity has also been shown to increase with training in rat heart and himdlimb muscles (Sen et al. 1992). An enhanced hepatic synthesis and output, coupled with a more vigorous transport, result in higher levels of GSH in the organs. Recent research suggests that GSH: GSSG homeostasis is a key factor in muscle inflammation and other pathogenic conditions associated with aging. For example, high levels of GSH prevent inflammatory process partially by inhibiting VCAM-1 expression (Kevil et al. 2004). Interestingly, oxidants (such as menadione) could only transiently decrease GSH levels in the endothelium, as GSH content measured 6–12 h after withdrawal of the oxidant stress increased by twofold accompanied by a twofold increase in GCS activity and 1.3–1.6-fold increase in GCS mRNA expression (Ray et al. 2002). GSH content was also reported to be higher in rabbit tibialis muscle 24 h after an isokinetic stretch injury, accompanied with elevated GPX and GR activities (Best et al. 1999).

Adaptation of body immune system to exercise may have a mixed impact on the oxidative stress level at senescence (Gleeson et al. 2006; Petersen and Pedersen

2006). Training has been shown to attenuate circulatory levels of pro-inflammatory cytokines such as TNFα, IL-1 and 6. Higher levels of habitual physical activity are associated with lower mitogen-stimulated inflammatory cytokine production and lower levels of skeletal muscle inflammatory protein. This suppression is a huge benefit for reducing oxidative stress and cell damage, since aging is often associated with a chronic low level inflammation especially in aged skeletal muscle due to minor injury and/or immobility (Bar-Shai et al. 2005). NFκB is believed to be constitutively activated at old age, which leads to the higher basal expression of pro-inflammatory cytokines, chemokines, adhesion molecules (ICAM-1, VCAM) and ROS-generating enzymes (iNOS and COX-2). In fact, chronic activation of NFκB has been identified as a main etiological reason for aged-related muscle wasting and sarcopenia (Cai et al. 2004). Yu and Chung (2006) demonstrated that 4-hydoxyhenxenal, a lipid peroxidation product often found in aged muscle, could activate NFκB by activating NIK/IKK signaling cascade due to ERK and p38 activation. Since NFκB activation often leads to increased pro-inflammatory cytokine expression, this vicious cycle was hypothesized as the basis for the inflammation theory of aging.

It is noteworthy that the hormetic effect of exercise on inducing antioxidant defense and reducing oxidative damage can be accomplished only at moderate, but not damaging intensity. "Non-damaging" is important but difficult to define in absolute terms because it depends on many factors such as prior training level, gender, age and nutritional status. Generally, it means the oxidative-antioxidant homeostasis is not overwhelmed by ROS resulting in irreversible changes. Past research has well established that strenuous exercise could cause high levels of ROS generation associated with cell damage in the skeletal muscle, heart and liver. Many of the benefits mentioned in previous sections can be achieved by participating in mild to moderate intensity of exercise. Several recent studies in rodents showed that voluntary wheel running could elicit protective effects on mitochondrial biogenesis (Akimoto et al. 2005) and prevent apoptosis (Phillips and Leeuwenburgh 2005). In humans, few studies could document a significant training effect on antioxidant enzymes (Tonkonogi and Sahlin 2002). The variability of prior physical activity levels and the difficulty to obtain homogenous muscle biopsy samples are potential confounding factors.

Molecular Mechanism of Exercise-Induced Hormesis

Hormesis is a pharmacological term meaning low dosage of toxins may increase body's tolerance for greater toxicity (Finkel and Holbrook 2000). Exercise-induced hormetic effects are conferred primarily by an upregulation of antioxidant enzymes through redox signaling (Ji 2007). The key to understanding exercise-induced hormetic response lies on the fact that mammalian cells are endowed with signaling pathways that are sensitive to intracellular redox environment and can be activated by oxidative stress. Those include NFκB, heat-shock transcriptional factor 1 (HSF-1), and P53 pathways, as well as mitogen-activated protein kinase (MAPK) and PI(3)K/

Akt that regulate the first three pathways through phosphorylation. Although all of these pathways are important in regulating normal growth and metabolism, NFκB and MAPK are considered the most critical for the cells to cope with oxidative stress (Allen and Tresini 2000). An acute bout of exercise has been shown to activate MAPK and NFκB signal transduction pathways in both animal and human studies (Ji 2007). The three main MAPK pathways, JNK, ERK1/2 and $p38^{MAPK}$, were activated in rat skeletal muscle after an acute bout of treadmill running (Goodyear 1996). ERK1/2 was reportedly activated after bicycle exercise in human muscle, along with activation of MEK1 and Raf-1 (MEKK), two upstream enzymes controlling ERK, as well as downstream enzyme p90 ribosomal S6 kinase (RSK). The signals triggering the MAPK activation have been attributed to a variety of physiological stimuli associated with exercise including hormones, calcium ion, neural activity, and mechanical force. Biological implications of MAPK activation are widespread including such important functions as glucose transport, muscle and heart hypertrophy, angiogenesis, and vascular adaptation (Hawley and Zierath 2004; Sakamoto and Goodyear 2002).

NFκB is activated by a variety of external stimulants, such as H_2O_2, pro-inflammatory cytokines (TNF-α, IL-1, IL-6), lipopolysaccharide (LPS), phorboester PMA, ionizing irradiation, and viral infection (Baeuerle and Baltimore 1988; Li and Karin 1999). These signals result in the phosphorylation and activation of IκB kinase (IKK) which phosphorylates two critical serine residues in IκB and primes IκB for ubiquitination and proteolytic degradation by the 26S proteasome. IκB dissociation unleashes P50/P65 to dimerize and translocate into the nucleus and bind the κB consensus sequence of the target genes. During and shortly after an acute bout of prolonged exercise, NFκB and AP-1 binding was significantly elevated in rat skeletal muscle in a fiber-specific manner (Hollander et al. 2001; Ji et al. 2004; Ho et al. 2005). NFκB binding was accompanied with increased IKK activity, IκB phosphorylation and degradation, and P50 nuclear translocation. These findings were confirmed in several different muscle fibers such as DVL, soleus and red gastrocnemius. Time course studies reveal that IKK activation and IkB phosphorylation could occur as early as 15–60 min, whereas P50/65 nuclear translocation and maximal NFκB binding was at 2–3 h. Noticeably, application of p38 and ERK inhibitors reduced IKK activation, suggesting MAPK and NFκB might work synergistically during exercise (Ho et al. 2005). The reliance of NFκB activation on MAPK is probably explained by the fact that NFκB activating kinase (NIK) is a member of MEKK family. Li and Engelhardt (2006) reported that IL-1β stimulation of NFκB is partially regulated by H_2O_2 -induced activation of NIK due to the inhibition of NIK phosphatase with the oxidation of a critical cysteine residue. Interestingly, activation of NIK can only be conferred within a narrow range of H_2O_2 concentration of 1–10 μM, close to physiological range within the cell.

Activation of redox-sensitive signaling pathways are overtures to upregulation of gene expression of antioxidant enzymes and other important proteins for the maintenance of oxidant-antioxidant homeostasis, which is deemed essential during aging. Some of these proteins may be double-edged sword, i.e., whereas adequate levels of expression offer extra protections, excessive expression may exacerbate oxidative stress. Several major gene targets of antioxidant signaling are introduced below.

MnSOD MnSOD promoter contains NFκB and AP-1 binding sites, which are sensitive to ROS, TNFα and IL-1 stimulation (Das et al. 1995). During heavy exercise, mitochondrial production of H_2O_2 is increased due to elevated ETC respiration. TNFα and IL-1 levels can also increase especially during strenuous muscle contraction and LC. These external stimuli may activate protein kinase C (PKC) and NIK as the distal key enzymes leading to the activation of NFκB cascades. However, even though NFκB binding at the promoter region constitutes a required condition, it does not guarantee a MnSOD upregulation. Jones et al. (1997) identified a 238-bp region of intron 2 that was responsive to TNFα and IL-1. This TNFα response element (TNFRE) contained both NFκB and 5′-CCAAT enhancer binding protein (C/EBP) motifs, shown to be both necessary and sufficient for TNF responsiveness. Guo et al. (2003) further explored the mechanism of MnSOD gene expression and elucidated two regulatory regions on MnSOD DNA, the proximal promoter region (PPR) and the above-mentioned TNFRE. Furthermore, MnSOD expression was shown to be activated by platelet-derived growth factor (PDGF) due to early growth-responsive-1 (egr-1) protein binding to a putative GC-rich region within the second intron of MnSOD gene, which may be controlled by MEK1 and ERK1/2 signaling (Maehara et al. 2001). Since MEK1 and ERK1/2 are activated in response to exercise, these regulatory sites may provide additional mechanisms for MnSOD transactivation. Indeed, ERK1/ERK2 and p38 ^{MAPK} activation was shown to accompany NFκB activation and a twofold increase in MnSOD mRNA level in rats subjected to an acute bout of progressive treadmill running (Gomez-Cabrera 2005). Figure 2 depicts the intracellular redox signaling pathways that potentially can induce MnSOD (For details see Ji 2007).

GPX GPX is a homotetramer with each 22-kDa subunit bound to a selenium atom existing as a selenocysteine (Holliwell and Gutteridge 1989). Two oxygen response elements (ORE) located at −1232 to −1213 and −282 to −275 in the 5′-flanking region of human GPX gene have been identified (Cowan et al. 1992). The expression of the GPX gene, *hgpx1*, occurs in a wide range of tissues controlled by development, hormones, and oxygen tension. In the myocardium, GPX activity induced by oxygen tension was found to be proportional to the mRNA levels, suggesting a transcriptional mechanism (Cowan et al. 1993). GPX promoter contains both NFκB and AP-1 binding sites. Zhou et al. (2001) showed that H_2O_2 and paraquat-induced GPX mRNA expression in C2C12 cell culture was dependent on functional NFκB signaling. Introduction of IκB mutant abolished GPX mRNA expression. Both cytosolic and mitochondrial fraction of GPX activity has also shown to increase after endurance training in skeletal muscle (Ji 1995). However, steady state GPX mRNA levels in trained rat muscles were found to be similar to those from the sedentary animals (Gore et al. 1998). Given the importance of GPX in muscle cells to remove H_2O_2 and lipid peroxide, more research is needed in elucidating GPX gene regulation in response to exercise.

GCS GSH plays a critical role in muscle antioxidant defense during exercise by providing substrate for GPX, maintaining proper redox status and scavenging $^{\bullet}OH$ and $O_2^{\bullet-}$. Surprisingly, little is known about the gene regulation of GCS in skeletal muscle. In mammalian cells, GCS is a heterodimer consisting of the catalytic

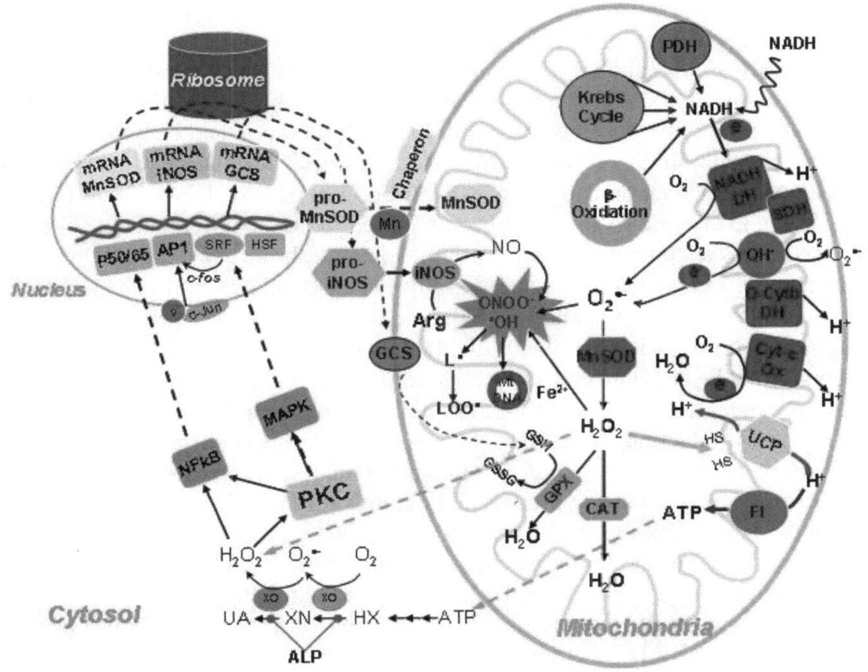

Fig. 2 The role of MnSOD and iNOS in mitochondrial antioxidant defense against oxidative damage and hypothetical signal transduction pathways of MnSOD and iNOS gene expression in the muscle cell. Abbreviations: 26S, 26S proteasome; CAT, catalase; GCS, γ-glumatylcysteine synthetase; GPX, glutathione peroxidase; HX, hypoxanthine; LOO•, lipid peroxyl radical; MEK, MAP/ERK kinase; MKK, MAP kinase kinase; Nox, NAPDH oxidase; PKC, protein kinase C; SDH, succinate dehydrogenase; QH•, ubisemiquinone; SRF, serum response factor; UA, uric acid; UCP, uncoupling protein. Other abbreviations: see text

heavy-chair subunit (GCS-HS) and regulatory light-chair subunit (GCS-LC) (Rahman and McNee 2000). GCS-HS expression is known to be regulated by redox-sensitive mechanism via a variety of oxidants, phenolic antioxidants and pro-inflammatory cytokines (TNFα and IL-1β). Both GCS-HC and GCS-LC promoters contain antioxidant response element (ARE) and NRF-2 binding seems to play a critical role in oxidative stress-induced GCS upregulation. GCS-HC also has NFκB binding sites that are essential for GCS expression in some, but not all cell types (Chan and Kwong 2000; Haddad 2002). If these signaling pathways are also operational in muscle cells, they could be potential mechanism for training-induced upregulation of GCS and GSH biosynthesis.

iNOS NO at low concentration exerts an antioxidant function by removing $O_2^{-\bullet}$ (Reid 2001). Its vasodilative effect increases blood flow to the working muscle thereby improving the availability of blood-borne energy substrates and antioxidants. Thus, an increase in NO production via the regulation of NOS may be viewed as indirectly enhancing muscle antioxidant defense during exercise. Unlike the other forms of NOS, iNOS is not regulated by calcium ion and instead responsive primarily to ROS and inflammatory cytokines through activation of NFκB and MAPK (Adams et al. 2002). In rat skeletal muscle myoblasts, the IL-1β-mediated iNOS induction was reduced by blocking ERK1/2 activation and completely abolished by the inhibition of NFκB. Moreover, a linear correlation was observed between NFκB activation and iNOS expression in human skeletal muscle (Adam et al. 2003). iNOS mRNA level has been reported to elevate after an acute bout of exercise in rat skeletal muscle (Balon 1999; Gomez-Cabrera et al. 2005). However, while chronic exercise training successfully increased nNOS and eNOS activity and protein expression, it failed to induce iNOS in rat gastrocnemius and diaphragm muscles (Vassilakopoulos et al. 2003). The role of iNOS is largely viewed as being catabolic and it is often co-expressed with pro-inflammatory cytokines and adhesion molecules during muscle injury and wasting (Schulze et al. 2002). High levels of NO production also lead to the formation of peroxynitrite, a highly reactive species contributing to muscle oxidative damage. Therefore, regulation of iNOS expression is a delicate process and requires further investigation.

Increased muscle mitochondrial number and protein may be the ultimate adaptation in reducing muscle oxidative stress, as postulated by Davies et al. (1982). Almost 3 decades ago, Chance et al. (1979) pointed out that cytochrome c oxidase might be considered the most important antioxidant enzyme as it secures electron flow to oxygen in ETC thereby decreasing potential formation of $O_2^{\bullet-}$. These foresights have been highlighted by the recent advances in studying exercise-induced mitochondrial biogenesis. The interactions of ROS, MAPK signaling and peroxisome proliferator-activated receptor-γ coactivator 1 (PGC-1), the master transcription factor of mitogenesis, have recently been shown to play a vital role in mitochondrial biogenesis of rodent muscle (Akimoto et al. 2005). Excitingly, PGC-1 expression has recently been shown to be associated with enhanced antioxidant gene expression and reduced oxidative stress (St-Pierre et al. 2006). It is not unthinkable that increased PGC-1 signaling may be instrumental in protecting skeletal muscle from sarcopenia.

Aging and Hormesis: A LifeTime Race

It has long been suspected that senescent skeletal muscle may compromise its ability to adapt to oxidative stress due to structural and functional impairment (Ji 2001; McArdle et al. 2002). Several relevant questions may be asked. (1) Does aged muscle have decreased level of protein components in the various redox signaling pathways? (2) Does aged muscle exhibit reduced sensitivity to oxidative challenge and diminished redox signaling potential? (3) What is the functional implication of this impairment and the potential strategy to reverse it? (4) Can exercise-induced hormetic effects be substituted by antioxidant supplementation? Due to the limited data available on this subject, only a few highlights will be mentioned. Readers are referred to several expert reviews for more insights (de Magalhaes and Church 2006; Yu and Chung 2006; Jackson 2005),

Hollander et al. (2000) reported NFκB and activating protein (AP)-1 binding at rest was attenuated in several types of skeletal muscle fibers of senescent rats. This led the authors to speculate that aging may attenuate cell's signal transduction capacity for antioxidant enzymes. This hypothesis was supported by other studies regarding NFκB activity in aged muscles (Radak et al. 2004). Broome et al. (2006) showed that NFκB binding was lower in senescent mouse muscle in response to stimulated contraction. Parkington et al. (2004) measured ERK1/2 and $p70^{S6K}$ activities in the plantaris and tibialis anterior muscles of young and old rats in response to electric stimulation and concluded that signaling of anabolic response to contractile stimulus is attenuated with aging, which may contribute to reduced exercise-induced muscle hypertrophy. In contrast, Hornberger et al. (2005) found no difference in p38, $p70^{S6K}$ and JNK2 activities in EDL muscle between young and old rats. Williamson et al. (2003) even reported higher resting activities of ERK ½, $p90^{RSK}$, $p38^{MAPK}$ and JNK/SAPK in the leg muscle of old compared to young men. However, aged muscles had decreased MAPK enzyme activities after an acute bout of resistance contraction, whereas young ones increased these enzyme activities. Total amount of protein expression in the MAPK pathway was found unaltered with age. The above discrepancies derived from different species and muscle types are not surprising as muscle antioxidant signaling is highly fiber specific due to differential intrinsic rate of ROS generation. Varied antioxidant defense capacity among different muscle types may also alter the sensitivity of cells to ROS. It is also possible that senescent muscles are often subjected to chronic inflammation and higher levels of pro-inflammatory cytokines may be a confounding factor. Thus, it is still premature to draw a conclusion as to how aging affects signaling and hormetic response to oxidative stress in skeletal muscle.

In conclusion, it can be said that ROS generated during muscle contraction either from mitochondrial respiratory chain or other oxidases play a critical role in muscle adaptation to exercise-induced oxidative stress by activating redox-sensitive signal transduction of antioxidant enzymes and other proteins vital to cell survival and functionality. NFκB and MAPK are two major signaling pathways that can be activated in response to ROS stimulation. These hormetic effects could be an important mechanism to protect senescent skeletal muscle which is subjected to increased intrinsic ROS generation and oxidative stress. However, there is a delicate balance between oxidative stress and muscle adaptability hinged on redox signaling in senescence. The word "mild" oxidative stress may be the key to achieving this balance.

References

Adams V, Nehrhoff B, Spate U, Linke A, Schulze PC, Baur A, Gielen S, Hambrecht R, and Schuler G. 2002. Induction of iNOS expression in skeletal muscle by IL-1beta and NFkappaB activation: an in vitro and in vivo study. Cardiovasc Res 54:95–104

Adams V, Spate U, Krankel N, Schulze PC, Linke A, Schuler G, and Hambrecht R. 2003. Nuclear factor-kappa B activation in skeletal muscle of patients with chronic heart failure: correlation with the expression of inducible nitric oxide synthase. Eur J Cardiovasc Prev Rehabil 10:273–277

Akimoto T, Pohnert SC, Li P, Zhang M, Gumbs C, Rosenberg PB, Williams RS, and Yan Z. 2005. Exercise stimulates Pgc-1alpha transcription in skeletal muscle through activation of the p38 MAPK pathway. J Biol Chem 280:19587–19593

Allen RG, and Tresini M. 2000. Oxidative stress and gene regulation. Free Rad Biol Med 28: 463–499

Aoi W, Naito Y, Takanami Y, Kawai Y, Sakuma K, Ichikawa H, Yoshida N, and Yoshikawa T. 2004. Oxidative stress and delayed-onset muscle damage after exercise. Free Radic Biol Med 37:480–487

Baeuerle PA, and Baltimore D. 1988. Activation of DNA-binding activity in an apparently cytoplasmic precursor of the NFκB transcriptiona factor. Cell 53: 211–217

Balon TW. 1999. Integrative biology of nitric oxide and exercise. Exerc Sport Sci Rev 27:219–253

Bar-Shai M, Carmeli E, and Reznick AZ. 2005. The role of NF-kappaB in protein breakdown in immobilization, aging, and exercise: from basic processes to promotion of health. Ann NY Acad Sci 1057:431–447

Bejma J, and Ji LL. 1999. Aging and acute exercise enhances free radical generation and oxidative damage in skeletal muscle. J Appl Physiol 87:465–470

Bejma J, Ramires P, and Ji LL. 2000. Free Radical Generation and Oxidative stress with aging and exercise: Differential effects in the myocardium and liver. Acta Physiol Scand 169:343–351

Best TM, Fiebig R, Corr DT, Brickson S, and Ji LL. 1999. Free radical activity and the response of antioxidant enzymes and glutathione following acute muscle stretch injury in rabbits. J Appl Physiol 87:74–82

Bowles DK, Farrar RP, and Starnes JW. 1992. Exercise training improves cardiac function after ischemia in the isolated, working rat heart. Am J Physiol 263:H804–H809

Broome CS, Kayani AC, Palomero J, Dillmann WH, Mestril R, Jackson MJ, and McArdle A. 2006. Effect of lifelong overexpression of HSP70 in skeletal muscle on age-related oxidative stress and adaptation after nondamaging contractile activity. FASEB J 20:1549–1551

Cai D, Frantz JD, Tawa NE Jr, Melendez PA, Oh BC, Lidov HG, Hasselgren PO, Frontera WR, Lee J, Glass DJ, and Shoelson SE. 2004. IKKbeta/NF-kappaB activation causes severe muscle wasting in mice. Cell 119:285–298

Cannon JG, and Blumberg JB. 1994. Acute phase immune responses in exercise, in Exercise and Oxygen Toxicity, edited by Sen CK, Packer L, Hanninen O. Elsevier Science, p. 447–479, New York

Chan JY, and Kwong M. 2000. Impaired expression of glutathione synthetic enzyme genes in mice with targeted deletion of the Nrf2 basic-leucine zipper protein. Biochim Biophys Acta 1517:19–26

Chance B, Sies H, and Boveris A. 1979. Hydroperoxide metabolism in mammalian organs. Physiol Rev 59:527–605

Chandwaney R, Leichtweis S, Leeuwenburgh C, and Ji LL. 1998. Oxidative stress and mitochondrial function in skeletal muscle: effects of aging and exercise training. Age 21: 109–117

Cowan DB, Weisel RD, Williams WG, and Mickle DAG. 1993. Identification of oxygen responsive elements in the 5″-flanking region of the human glutathione peroxidase gene. J Biol Chem 268:26904–26910

Cowan DB, Weisel RD, Williams WG, and Mickle DAG. 1992. The regulation of glutathione peroxidase gene expression by oxygen tension in cultured human cardiomyocytes. J Mol Cell Cardiol 24:423–433

Davies KJA, Quantanilla AT, Brooks GA, and Packer L. 1982. Free radicals and tissue damage produced by exercise. Biochem Biophys Res Comm 107:1198–1205

Das KC, Lewis-Molock Y, and White CW. 1995. Thiol modulation of TNF alpha and IL-1 induced MnSOD gene expression and activation of NF-kappa B. Mol Cell Biochem 148:45–57
de Magalhaes JP, and Church GM. 2006. Cells discover fire: employing reactive oxygen species in development and consequences for aging. Exp Gerontol 41:1–10
Droge W. 2006. Redox regulation in anabolic and catabolic processes. Curr Opin Clin Nutr Metab Care 9:190–195
Fiebig R, Leeuwenburgh C, Gore M, and Ji LL. 1996. The interactive effects of aging and training on myocardial antioxidant enzymes and oxidative stress. Age 19:83–89
Fries JF. 1996. Physical activity, the compression of morbidity, and the health of the elderly. J Royal Soc Med 89:64–68
Gath I, Closs EI, Godtel-Armburst U, Schmitt S, Nakane M, Wessler I, and Forestermann U. 1996. Inducible NO synthase II and neuronal NO synthase I are constitutively expressed in different structures of guinea pig skeletal muscle: implications for contractile function. FASEB J 10:1614–1620
Gleeson M, McFarlin B, and Flynn M. 2006. Exercise and Toll-like receptors. Exerc Immunol Rev 12:34–53
Gomez-Cabrera M-C, Borras C, Santangelo G, Pallardó FV, Sastre J, Ji LL, and Vina J. 2005. Decreasing xanthine oxidase mediated oxidative stress prevents useful cellular adatptations to exercise in rats. J Physiol (London) 567:113–120
Goodyear L, Chang P, Sherwood D, Dufresne S, and Moller D. 1996. Effects of exercise and insulin on mitogen-activated protein kinase signaling pathways in rat skeletal muscle. Am J Physiol 171:E403–E408
Gore M, Fiebig R, Hollander J, Griffiths M, Leeuwenburgh C, Ohno H, and Ji LL. 1998. Exercise training alters antioxidant enzyme gene expression in rat skeletal muscle. Can J Physiol Pharmacol 76:1139–1145
Goto S, Natio H, Kaneko T, Chung HY, and Rakak Z. 2007. Hormetic effects of regular exercise in aging: correlation with oxidative stress. Appl Physiol Nutr Met (in press)
Guo Z, Boekhoudt H, and Boss JM. 2003. Role of the intronic enhancer in tumor necrosis factor-mediated induction of manganous superoxide dismutase. J Biol Chem 278:23570–23578
Haddad JJ. 2002. The involvement of L-gamma-glutamyl-L-cysteinyl-glycine (glutathione/GSH) in the mechanism of redox signaling mediating MAPK(p38)-dependent regulation of pro-inflammatory cytokine production. Biochem Pharmacol 63:305–320
Halliwell B, and Gutteridge JMC. 1989. Free Radicals in Biology and Medicine. Clarendon, Oxford
Harman D. 1956. Aging: a theory based on free radical and radiation chemistry. J Gerontol 11:298–300
Hawley JA, and Zierath JR. 2004. Integration of metabolic and mitogenic signal transduction in skeletal muscle. Exerc Sport Sci Rev 32:4–8
Ho RC, Hirshman MF, Li Y, Cai D, Farmer JR, Aschenbach WG, Witczak CA, Shoelson SE, and Goodyear LJ. 2005. Regulation of IkappaB kinase and NF-kappaB in contracting adult rat skeletal muscle. Am J Physiol Cell Physiol 289:C794–C801
Hollander J, Bejma J, Ookawara T, Ohno H, and Ji LL. 2000. Superoxide dismutase gene expression in skeletal muscle: fiber-specific effect of age. Mech Age Dev 116:33–45
Hollander J, Fiebig R, Ookawara T, Ohno H, and Ji LL. 2001. Superoxide dismutate gene expression is activated by a single bout of exercise. Pflug Arch (Eur J Physiol) 442:426–434
Holluszy JO. 1993. Exercise increases average longevity of female rats despite increased food intake and no growth retardation. J Gerontol 48:B97–B100
Hornberger TA, Mateja RD, Chin ER, Andrews JL, and Esser KA. 2005. Aging does not alter the mechanosensitivity of the p38, p70S6k, and JNK2 signaling pathways in skeletal muscle. J Appl Physiol 98:1562–1566
Jackson M. 2005. Reactive oxygen species and redox-regulation of skeletal muscle adaptations to exercise. Phil Trans R Soc B 360:2285–2291
Ji LL. 1995. Exercise and oxidative stress: role of the cellular antioxidant systems. In Holloszy, JO (Ed.). Exercise Sports Science Reviews, pp. 135–166, Williams & Wilkins, Baltimore, MD

Ji LL. 1999. Antioxidants and oxidative stress in exercise. Proc Soc Exp Biol Med 222:283–292

Ji LL. 2001. Exercise at old age: does it increase or alleviate oxidative stress? Ann NY Acad Sci 923:236–247

Ji LL. 2007. Antioxidant signaling in skeletal muscle: a brief review. Exp Gerontol 42:582–593

Ji LL, Dillon D, and Wu E. 1990. Alteration of antioxidant enzymes with aging in rat skeletal muscle and liver. Am J Physiol 258:R918–R923

Ji LL, Gomez-Cabrera M-C, Steinhafel N, and Vina J. 2004. Acute exercise activates nuclear factor (NF) κB signaling pathway in rat skeletal muscle. FASEB J 18:1499–1506

Jones PL, Ping D, and Boss JM. 1997. Tumor necrosis factor alpha and interleukin-1beta regulate the murine manganese superoxide dismutase gene through a complex intronic enhancer involving C/EBP-beta and NF-kappaB. Mol Cell Biol 17:6970–6981

Kevil CG, Pruitt H, Kavanagh TJ, Wilkerson J, Farin F, Moellering D, Darley-Usmar VM, Bullard DC, and Patel RP. 2004. Regulation of endothelial glutathione by ICAM-1: implications for inflammation. FASEB J 18:1321–1323

Kim JD, McCarter RJM, and Yu BP. 1996. Influence of age, exercise, and dietary restriction on oxidative stress in rats. Aging Clin Exp Res 8:123–129

Lawler JM, Powers SK, Visser T, Van Dijk H, Korthuis MJ, and Ji LL. 1993. Acute exercise and skeletal muscle antioxidant and metabolic enzymes: effect of fiber type and age. Am J Physiol 265:R1344–R1350

Leeuwenburgh C, Hansen PA, Holloszy JO, and Heinecke JW. 1999. Hydroxyl radical generation during exercise increases mitochondrial protein oxidation and levels of urinary dityrosine. Free Radic Biol Med 27:186–192

Leeuwenburgh, C, Fiebig, R, Chandwaney, R, and Ji, LL. 1994. Aging and exercise training in skeletal muscle: response of glutathione and antioxidant enzyme systems. Am J Physiol 267: R439–R445.

Li N, and Karin M. 1999. Is NFκB the sensor of oxidative stress? FASEB J 13:1137–1143

Li Q, and Engelhardt JF. 2006. Interlecukin-1β induction of NFκB is partially regulated by H_2O_2-mediated activation of NFκB-inducing kinase. J Biol Chem 281:1495–1505

Luhtala TA, Roecker EB, Pugh T, Feuers RJ, and Weindruch R. 1994. Dietary restriction attenuates age-related increases in rat skeletal muscle antioxidant enzyme activities. J Gerontol 49: B321–B328

Maehara K, Oh-Hashi K, and Isobe K-I. 2001. Early growth-responsive-1-dependent manganese superoxide dismutase gene transcript mediated by platelet-derived growth factor. FASEB J 15:2025–2026

Matsuo M. 1993. Age-related alterations in antioxidant defense. In Yu, BP (Ed.). Free Radicals in Aging, pp. 143–181). CRC, Boca Raton, FL

McArdle A, Vasilaki A, and Jackson M. 2002. Exercise and skeletal muscle ageing: cellular and molecular mechanisms. Ageing Res Rev 1:79–93

McArdle A, and Jackson MJ. 2000. Exercise, oxidative stress and ageing. J Anat 197: 539–541

McArdle A, Pattwell D, Vasilaki A, Griffiths RD, and Jackson MJ. 2001. Contractile activity-induced oxidative stress: cellular origin and adaptive responses. Am J Physiol 280: C621–C627

Meister A, and Anderson ME. 1983. Glutathione. Ann Rev Biochem 52:711–760

Meydani M, and Evans WJ. 1993. Free radicals, exercise, and aging. In Yu, BP (Ed.). Free Radical in Aging, pp. 183–204. CRC, Boca Raton, FL

Meydani M, and Evans WJ. 1993. Free radicals, exercise, and aging. In Yu, BP (Ed.). Free Radical in Aging, pp. 183–204. CRC, Boca Raton, FL

Nohl H, Breuninger V, and Hegner D. 1978. Influence of mitochondrial radical formation on energy-linked respiration. Eur J Biochem 90:385–390

Paffenbarger RS, Hyde RT, Wing AL, Lee IM, Jung DL, and Kampert JBG. 1993. The association of changes in physical activity level and other lifestyle characteristics with mortality among men. N Eng J Med 328:538–545

Pamplona R, Portero-Otin M, Requena JR, Herrero A, and Barja G. 1999. A low degree of fatty acid unsaturation leads to low lipid peroxidation lipoxidation-derived protein modification in heart mitochondria of the longeous pigeon than in the short-lived rat. Mech Age Dev 106:283–296

Parkington JD, LeBrasseur NK, Siebert AP, and Fielding RA. 2004. Contraction-mediated mTOR, p70S6k, and ERK1/2 phosphorylation in aged skeletal muscle. J Appl Physiol 97:243–248

Pattwell DM, McArdle A, Morgan A, Pateridge TA, and Jackson MJ. 2004. Release of reactive oxygen and nitrogen species from contracting skeletal muscle cells. Free Radic Biol Med 37:1064–1072

Pedersen BK, Ostrowski K, Rohde T, and Rruunsgaard H. 1998. The cytokine response to strenuous exercise. Can J Physiol Pharmacol 76:505–511

Petersen AM, and Pedersen BK. 2006. The role of IL-6 in mediating the anti-inflammatory effects of exercise. J Physiol Pharmacol 57 (Suppl. 10):43–51

Phillips T, and Leeuwenburgh C. 2005. Muscle fiber specific apoptosis and TNF-alpha signaling in sarcopenia are attenuated by life-long calorie restriction. FASEB J 19:668–670

Powers SK, Ji LL, and Leeuwenburgh C. 1999. Exercise training-induced antioxidant capacity: a brief review. Med Sci Sports Exer 31:987–997

Pyne DB. 1994. Regulation of neutrophil function during exercise. Sports Med. 17:245–258

Radak Z, Chung HY, Naito H, Takahashi R, Jung KJ, Kim HJ, and Goto S. 2004. Age-associated increase in oxidative stress and nuclear factor kappaB activation are attenuated in rat liver by regular exercise. FASEB J 18:749–750

Rahman I, and MacNee W. 2000. Oxidative stress and regulation of glutathione in lung inflammation. Eur Respir J 16:534–554

Ray S, Watkins DN, Misso NL, and Thompson PJ. 2002. Oxidant stress induces gamma-glutamylcysteine synthetase and glutathione synthesis in human bronchial epithelial NCI-H292 cells. Clin Exp Allergy 32:571–577

Reid MB. 2001. Redox modulation of skeletal muscle contraction: what we know and what we don't. J Appl Physiol 90:724–731

Reid MB. 2001. Redox modulation of skeletal muscle contraction: what we know and what we don't. J Appl Physiol 90:724–731

Sakamoto K, and Goodyear LJ. 2002. Invited review: intracellular signaling in contracting skeletal muscle. J Appl Physiol 93:369–383

Sakurai T, Hollander J, Brickson S, Izawa T, Ohno H, Ji LL, and Best TM. 2005. Changes in nitric oxide and inducible nitric oxide synthase following stretch-induced injury to the tibialis anterio muscle of rabbit. Japan J Physiol 55:101–107

Sawada M, Sester U, and Carlson JC. 1992. Superoxide radical formation and associated biochemical alterations in the plasma membrane of brain, heart, and liver during the lifetime of the rat. J Cell Biochem 48:296–304

Schulze PC, Gielen S, Schuler G, and Hambrecht R. 2002. Chronic heart failure and skeletal muscle catabolism: effects of exercise training. In J Cardiol 85:141–149

Sen CK. 1995. Oxidants and antioxidants in exercise. J. Appl. Physiol. 79:675–686

Sen CK, Marin E, Kretzschmar M, and Hanninen O. 1992. Skeletal muscle and liver glutathione homeostasis in response to training, exercise, and immobilization. J Appl Physiol 73:1265–1272

Sohal RS, and Sohal BH. 1991. Hydrogen peroxide release by mitochondria increases during aging. Mech Age Dev 57:187–202

St-Pierre J, Drori S, Uldry M, Silvaggi JM, Rhee J, Jager S, Handschin C, Zheng K, Lin J, Yang W, Simon K, Bachoo R, and Spiegelman BM. 2006. Suppression of reactive oxygen species and neurodegeneration by the PGC-1 transcriptional coactivators. Cell 127:397–408

Thomas DR. 2007. Loss of skeletal muscle mass in aging: examining the relationship of starvation, sarcopenia and cachexia. Clin Nutr (in press, www.sciencedirect.com)

Titball JG, Lavergne E, Lau KS, Spencer MJ, Stull JT, and Wehling M. 1998. Mechanical loading regulates NOS expression and activity in developing and adult skeletal muscle. Am J Phsiol 275:C260–C266

Tonkonogi M, and Sahlin K. 2002. Physical exercise and mitochondrial function in human skeletal muscle. Exerc Sport Sci Rev 30:129–137

Vassilakopoulos T, Deckman G, Kebbewar M, Rallis G, Harfouche R, and Hussain SN. 2003. Regulation of nitric oxide production in limb and ventilatory muscles during chronic exercise training. Am J Physiol Lung Cell Mol Physiol 284:L452–L457

Williamson D, Gallagher P, Harber M, Hollon C, and Trappe S. 2003. Mitogen-activated protein kinase (MAPK) pathway activation: effects of age and acute exercise on human skeletal muscle. J Physiol 547:977–987

Yu BP, and Chung HY. 2006. Adaptive mechanisms to oxidative stress during aging. Mech Age Dev 127:436–443

Zhou LZ, Johnson AP, and Rando TA. 2001. NF kappa B and AP-1 mediate transcriptional responses to oxidative stress in skeletal muscle cells. Free Radic Biol Med 31:1405–1416

Chapter 8
How Xenohormetic Compounds Confer Health Benefits

Brian J. Morris[1]

Introduction

Compounds that are capable of inducing damage to cells, so leading the cells to activate defence pathways to protect the cell, have been referred to as 'hormetins' (Ali and Rattan 2006). Then there is the situation whereby natural environmental stresses stimulate plants to produce specific endogenous chemicals that help protect the plant against the change in conditions that could otherwise be detrimental. These are regarded as 'hormetic compounds'. Animals that live in the same locality are also under selective pressure to develop protective mechanisms to assist in their survival in the face of the same environmental change. The xenohormesis hypothesis (Lamming et al. 2004) proposes that organisms have evolved to respond to stress signalling molecules ('hormetic' compounds) produced by dietary plant species where they live, so enabling them to be prepared to resist potentially detrimental effects. Under stressful conditions such as cold or drought, when plants ramp up their production of these specialized chemical compounds, by eating the plants, the benefit is transferred to animals. The plant chemicals, when acting on animals in this way, can be referred to as xenohormetic compounds, and are the focus of this chapter. It is indeed quite intriguing that animals have evolved mechanisms to utilize these same plant compounds consumed in their diet. Even more fascinating is that this leads to the activation of similar protective mechanisms in the cells of the animals as are activated in the cells of the plants.

The Mediterranean diet is one good example. To protect themselves from environmental stress, plants such as the grape vine and olive trees in the Mediterranean basin, have developed an array of antioxidant defences. The Mediterranean diet is renowned for its health benefits. The people in this region of the world traditionally exhibit lower rates of coronary heart disease and certain cancers. Apart from the

[1]School of Medical Sciences, Building F13, The University of Sydney, New South Wales 2006, Australia.

Address for correspondence:
Professor Brian J. Morris, School of Medical Sciences and Bosch Institute, Building F13, The University of Sydney, Sydney, New South Wales 2006, Australia. Tel: +61-2-93513688; Fax: +61-2-93512227; e-mail: brianm@medsci.usyd.edu.au

E. Le Bourg and S.I.S. Rattan (eds.), *Mild Stress and Healthy Aging*.

health benefits of the monounsaturated oil in olive oil, 1–2% of cold-pressed extra virgin olive oil contains polyphenols, tocopherols, sterols, triterpenoids, hydrocarbons, and traces of other compounds that have antioxidant, anti-inflammatory and hypolipidaemic properties (Perona et al. 2006). Deposition of plaque in the endothelium of blood vessels is the hallmark of atherosclerosis. These compounds, in large part by activating nuclear factor κB (NF-κB), modulate the production of vasodilators, nitric oxide (NO) and eicosanoids, such as prostaglandins and leukotrienes, as well as adhesion molecules involved in the atherosclerotic process (Perona et al. 2006). The polyphenols hydroxytyrosol and oleuropein are potent scavengers of reactive oxygen species (ROS). At 10^{-5} M, oleuropein prevents oxidative damage to low density lipoprotein (LDL) (Visioli and Galli 1994). These various actions help explain, at least in part, why the Mediterranean diet protects from atherosclerosis.

Food Shortage – A Hormetic Stress

One of the most common environmental stressors is food shortage. This activates various pathways in the cells of animals to help them resist the food shortage and protect the animal until such time as food returns (Morris 2005). One obvious effect is suppression of reproduction, as this would obviously be undesirable when food is scarce. By lengthening lifespan under conditions of caloric reduction the animal is more likely to survive longer. Once the food supply has returned reproduction can be switched on again. Calorie restriction activates sirtuin-mediated signalling pathways such as those involving insulin, so explaining the opposite effects on lifespan extension/survival versus reproduction (Morris 2005).

The activation of sirtuin pathways is highly conserved through evolution and has been found to increase the lifespan of diverse organisms. Such effects are most pronounced, however, for animals with shorter lifespans. By restricting caloric intake by 30–40% while maintaining adequate nutrient intake the lifespan of nematodes can be increased several fold, the fruit fly 70%, whereas in rats calorie restriction adds 30% to the lifespan (McCay et al. 1935; Guarente and Kenyon 2000; Everitt 2003; Koubova and Guarente 2003). The *Drosophila* data have, however, been criticized, so that this finding remains inconclusive, with some believing that animals with the ability to flee an adverse environment may not have needed to evolve mechanisms to extend lifespan (Le Bourg and Minois 2005).

In humans, caloric restriction confers health benefits consistent with reduced risk of cardiovascular and other diseases (Walford et al. 2002; Fontana et al. 2004). The first person to deliberately set out to demonstrate the efficacy of caloric restriction was Luigi Cornano (Turner 2003). He began food restriction at age 40 and lived a ripe old age, reported variously as 89 through 102 years, which, irrespective, is quite old today, let alone for the 15th century! No population studies exist at present to prove that calorie restriction is indeed able to increase human lifespan. Based on sound arguments for or against this possibility, the various experts in the field remain divided (Le Bourg and Rattan 2006). Most agree, however, that calorie restriction should increase 'health span'.

Interestingly, the pathways in the cell that are activated by caloric restriction are similarly activated by hormetic compounds. A modest, healthy diet rich in hormetic compounds may be able to achieve a similar outcome as calorie restriction. Consumption of these therefore represents a preferable alternative to most people, who would find calorie restriction difficult to maintain. Hormetic compounds may thus be regarded as calorie restriction mimetics. As can be seen in Fig. 1, both caloric restriction and hormetic compounds stimulate sirtuin enzymes in the cells, and this then leads to the activation of the various downstream pathways that aid in stress resistance.

Hormetic Compounds Are Common in Plants

Hormetic compounds are present in all vegetables and fruit, but the levels vary for different types and different growing conditions. Consequently claims abound about which ones to choose to maximize intake. Among the most well known are various berry fruit, broccoli, cocoa and green tea, but there are plenty of others. Stress, such as conferred by cold conditions, may result in higher levels of these in accord with the hormesis hypothesis. But hormetic compounds are present in plants, so that an increase in levels conferred by stress is not an absolute requirement for plants to be able to provide humans with an adequate intake of these.

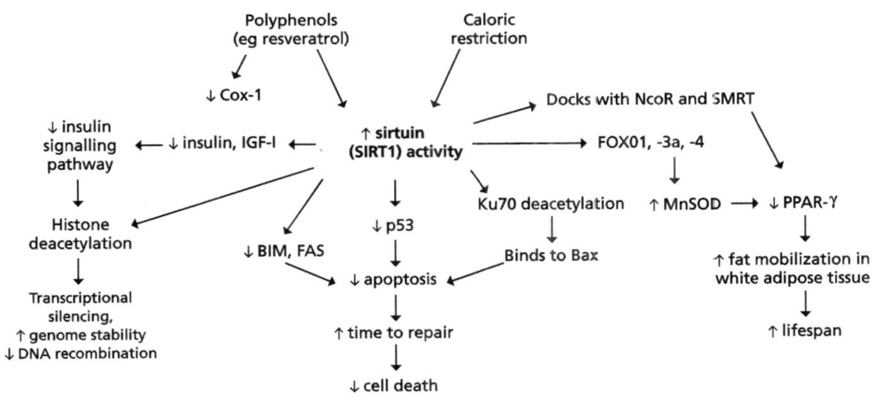

Fig. 1 Common pathways by which calorie restriction and polyphenols such as resveratrol enhance stress resistance and thus survival pathways in cells via stimulation of sirtuins. Abbreviations: Cox-1, cyclooxygenase-1; IGF-I, insulin-like growth factor-I; NcoR, nuclear receptor co-repressor; SMRT, silencing mediator of retinoid and thyroid hormone receptors; FOXO, forkhead/winged helix box gene, group O; SOD, superoxide dismutase; PPAR, peroxisome proliferator-activated receptor (Modified from Morris 2005)

Polyphenols

Polyphenols are natural constituents of vegetables, fruit, nuts, olive oil and various beverages. Preparations of seeds from the tree *Ginkgo biloba* are also a well-known source. Polyphenols can be grouped into tannins, lignins and flavonoids. The flavonoids are the largest category of polyphenols, and are made up the subclasses flavones, flavanones, isoflavones, flavonols and flavans. The average daily intake of flavonoids in food is 50–800 mg, depending on a person's dietary intake of different foods.

Phenolic compunds have anti-inflammatory effects. They reduce expression of adhesion molecules and cytokines as well as increasing endothelial nitric oxide synthase (eNOS) activity to raise NO release (Jiang and Dusting 2003). This action contributes to their ability to reduce the risk of cardiovascular disease. The antioxidant properties of polypenols, carotenoids such as lycopene and β-carotene, and coenzyme Q10 help in prevention of atherosclerosis (Kaliora et al. 2006). This involves reduction in the oxidation of LDL, as well as other actions (Fig. 2). Various kinds of these 'neutraceuticals' also help in the prevention and treatment of hypertension (Houston 2005). The flavonoid quercetin lowers blood pressure by causing vasodilatation of resistance vessels. It does this by stimulating eNOS and decreasing NADPH oxidase-mediated production of superoxide associated with reduced $p47^{phox}$ (Sánchez et al. 2006). Cocoa, which is rich in these compounds,

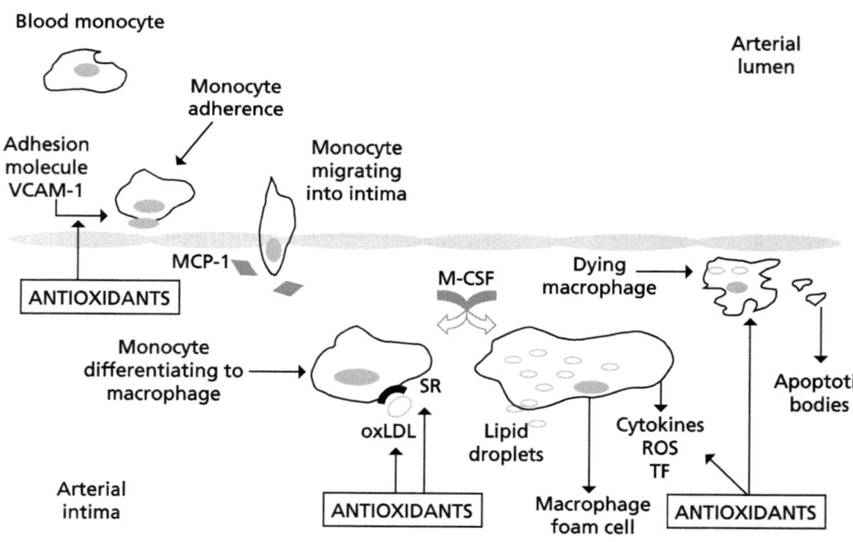

Fig. 2 How antioxidants, including flavanols, may affect atherogenesis. Abbreviations: MCP-1, monocyte chemoattractant protein-1; MCSF, macrophage colony stimulating factor; oxLDL, oxidized low density lipoprotein; TF, tissue factor; VCAM, vascular endothelial cell adhesion molecule (Modified from Kaliora et al. 2006)

stimulates vascular NO production leading to vasodilatation (Fisher et al. 2003). This is sufficient to explain the absence of hypertension in the Kuna Indians of Panama (McCullough et al. 2006). The benefits of cocoa may extend to prevention of atherosclerosis, type 2 diabetes, preeclampsia, vascular dementias and end-stage renal disease (Hollenberg 2006).

The antioxidant and other effects of polyphenols confer neuroprotection in models of Alzheimer's, Parkinson's and Huntington's disease (Mandel et al. 2005). Indeed, the glycosides and terpenoids (ginkgolides, bilobalides) in extracts of Ginkgo leaves are used pharmaceutically. Ginkgo extract appears to improve blood flow to tissues, protects against damage to cells from ROS, and blocks many of the effects of platelet activating factor, such as platelet aggregation and blood clotting, that would otherwise predispose to the development of cardiovascular, renal, respiratory and CNS disorders (Christen and Maixent 2002; Smith et al. 2002; Zimmermann et al. 2002; Christen 2004; Loh et al. 2006).

Tea Catechins

Fresh leaves from the tea plant (*Camellia sinensis*) contain high levels of the flavonoids or flavanols known as catechins. Green tea is a particularly rich source of catechins, notably (–)-epigallocetechin-3-gallate (EGCG), and related polyphenols (Fig. 3), which represent 30–45% of solid extracts (Wang et al. 1994). Catechins and their derivatives act directly as scavengers of ROS, and indirectly via activation of transcription factors and antioxidant enzymes (Higdon and Frei 2003). Relative antioxidant activities among tea catechins are: EGCG = (–)-epicatechin-3-gallate (ECG) > (–)-epigallocatechin (EGC) > (–)-epicatechin (EC) (Guo et al. 1999). These compounds not only scavenge ROS, but chelate metals via the 3',4'-dihydroxyl group in the B ring (Hider et al. 2001) and gallate group (Guo et al. 1996). This may neutralize ferric iron by converting it to iron, which is inactive, so protecting cells from oxidative damage (Grinberg et al. 1997). These are but some of the wide diversity of actions of catechins that enhance cell survival (Mandel et al. 2005). Indeed, catechins and other flavonoids have great potential for the treatment of the various amyloid diseases. For example, EGCG can reduce misfolding and oligomerization of mutant huntingtin and prevented the neural defects in transgenic *Drosophila* overexpressing this mutant protein (Ehrnhoefer et al. 2006).

EGCG has potential, moreover, as an antidiabetic agent. It has insulin-like properties by being able to lower glucose (Kao et al. 2000). EGCG and ECG inhibit glutamate dehydrogenase to modulate insulin secretion (Li et al. 2006). EGCG does this by inducing phosphatidyl kinase-3 mediated phosphorylation of insulin-sensitive residues on the forkhead/winged helix box, group O transcription factor FOXO1a, leading to repression of enzymes, such as the rate-limiting enzyme phosphoenolpyruvate carboxykinase, that are involved in gluconeogenesis (Anton et al. 2006). Unlike insulin, EGCG's induction of FOXO1a is sensitive to ROS.

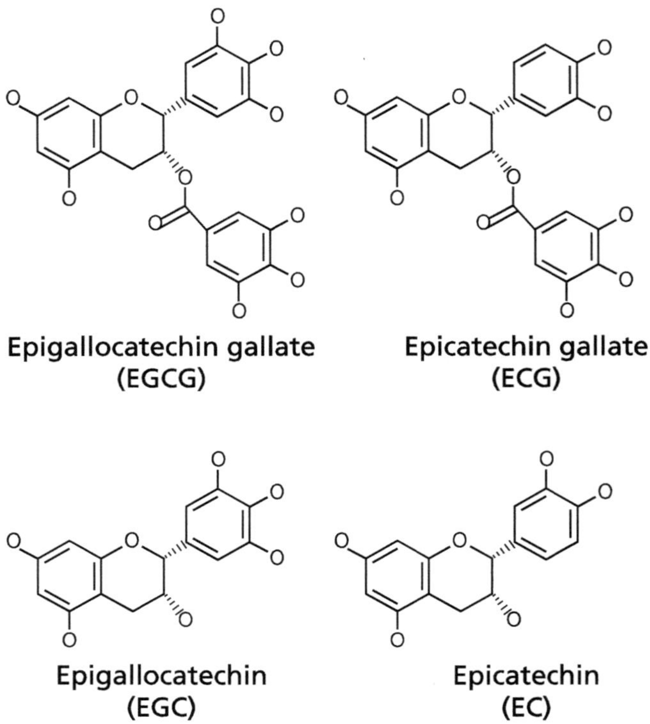

Fig. 3 Chemical structures of catechins and derivatives in green tea

In relation to hypertension, tea flavonoids reduce the risk of cardiovascular disease by improving endothelial function and possibly lowering blood pressure (Hodgson 2006).

Drinking green tea is inversely associated with several types of human cancer (Park and Surh 2004). Lower rates of breast and prostate cancer in Asian populations have been attributed to EGCG in tea (Park and Surh 2004). EGCG inhibits the proliferation of melanoma, breast cancer, lung cancer, leukaemia and colon cancer cell lines (Lambert and Yang 2003). Doses of approx ten times that seen after tea drinking inhibit mitogen-activated protein kinases, cyclin-dependent kinases, growth factor-related cell signalling, activation of activator protein 1 (AP-1) and NF-κB, topoisomerase I and matrix metalloproteinases, as well as other potential targets (Lambert and Yang 2003). Constitutive expression of cyclooxygenase 2 (Cox-2), which has a critical role in colon cancer, is inhibited by EGCG via inhibition of NF-κB activation (Peng et al. 2006). EGCG binds to DNA and RNA (Kuzuhara et al. 2006). This would explain why EGCG protects DNA from damage induced by ROS, ionizing radiation and ultraviolet light, and also from DNA methylation (Fang et al. 2003). The association of green tea consumption and cancer prevention is thus backed up by molecular changes observed in cells as a result of its constituent hormetic compounds (Fujiki 2005).

Genistein

Genistein (4'5, 7-trihydroxyisoflavone) is the most abundant isoflavone in soy products (2–200 µg/g) and may reduce risk of coronary heart disease and cancer (Cassidy 2003). It is safe, even at the high concentrations used in cancer trials (Bloedon et al. 2002; Busby et al. 2002). Genistein's consumption in a high soy diet has been implicated in lower rates of breast and prostate cancer in Asia in particular (Park and Surh 2004). It can also augment the efficacy of radiation therapy for these cancers (Ravindranath et al. 2004). By stimulating melanin production and tyrosinase activity, genistein can protect melanocytes from melanoma induced by UV-B radiation and also reduces melanoma incidence (Ravindranath et al. 2004).

Genistein can arrest cell growth and proliferation, cell cycle progression at the G2/M stage, tumour invasion and angiogenesis (Sarkar and Li 2002; Ravindranath et al. 2004). It does this by blocking the activities of protein tyrosine kinase, topoisomerase II and matrix metalloprotein-9, as well as by down-regulating the expression at least 11 genes including that for vascular endothelial growth factor (VEGF) (Ravindranath et al. 2004). As well, genistein alters the expression of gangliosides and other carbohydrate antigens to facilitate their immune recognition. Genistein acts synergistically with drugs such as tamoxifen, cisplatin, dexamethasone, and others, as well as with other flavonoids such as quercetin, green-tea catechins and black-tea thearubigins (Ravindranath et al. 2004).

Drinking soy milk for an extended period lowers blood pressure of people with mild to moderate essential hypertension (Rivas et al. 2002). At concentrations that can be achieved physiologically, genistein alters expression in human vascular endothelial cells of genes involved in control of blood pressure, such as endothelin converting enzyme-1, endothelin-2, oestrogen receptor-α and atrial natriuretic factor receptor A precursor (Ambra et al. 2006). It also counters the effect of oxidized LDL on expression of vascular endothelial growth factor receptor 165, types 1 and 2. These actions help explain its beneficial effects on the blood vessel wall.

Genistein strongly and selectively binds to and inhibits transthyretin in plasma, as well as transthyretin's disease-associated genetic variants, so reducing by over 90% the ability of each to induce amyloid fibril formation *in vitro* (Green et al. 2005). This may explain why it is an exceptional inhibitor of transthyretin amyloidogenesis, where senile systemic amyloidosis is characterized by the deposition of transthyretin in the heart and peripheral nerves. Genistein has undergone or is currently under clinical trial for treatment of breast, prostate and uterine cancers, osteoporosis, cardiovascular disease and menopausal symptoms.

Soy isoflavones also have a mild, but significant effect on bone mineral content in postmenopausal women with low bone mass (Chen et al. 2003).

Resveratrol – The Quintessential Hormetic Compound

One of the most potent hormetic compounds is the polyphenolic flavonoid, resveratrol (also known as either *trans*-3,5,4′-trihydroxystilbene or 5-[(E)-2-(4-hydroxyphenyl)-ethenyl]benzene-1,3-diol; $C_{14}H_{12}O_3$) (Fig. 4), found in grape skins and seeds, red wine, mulberries, peanuts and rhubarb. Of various small molecule sirtuin activators tested, resveratrol is the most potent (Howitz et al. 2003). Consistent with the hormesis hypothesis, levels of polyphenols are elevated in cultivars of *Vitis vinifera* when growing conditions are harsher (Morris 2007).

Cardiovascular Protection

Various epidemiological studies suggest that red wine and grape extracts might confer additional benefits to alcohol alone (Bohm et al. 2004). These include a reduction in platelet aggregation, dilatation of blood vessels, anti-atherosclerotic

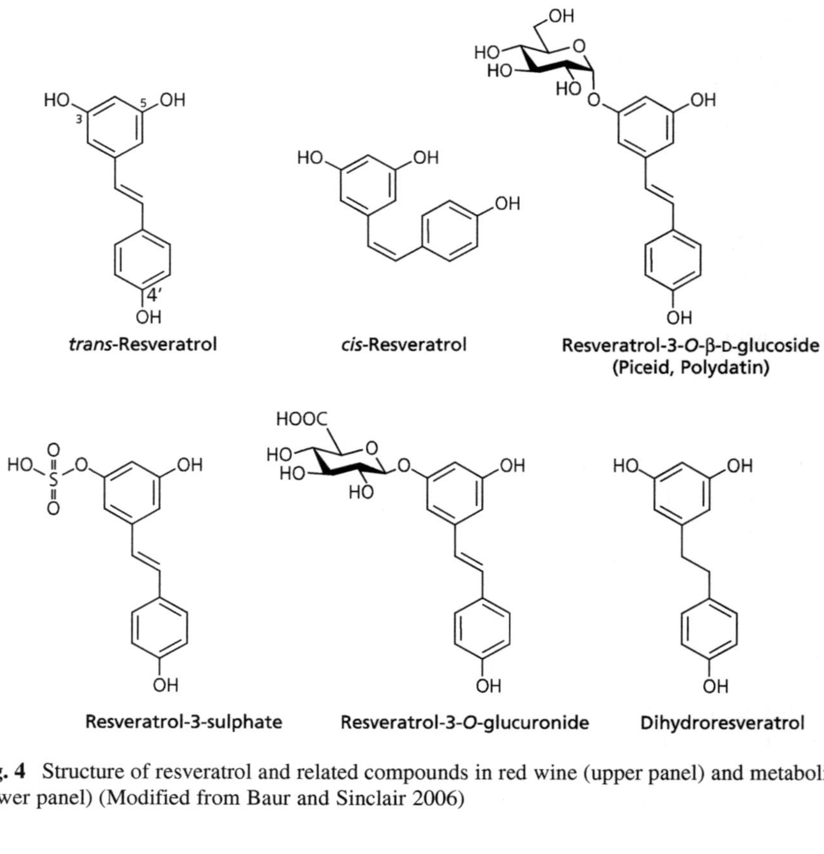

Fig. 4 Structure of resveratrol and related compounds in red wine (upper panel) and metabolites (lower panel) (Modified from Baur and Sinclair 2006)

effects, lowering of lipid peroxidation, reduction in endothelin-1, protection of endothelial cells against apoptosis, lowering of blood pressure, oxidative stress and end-organ damage in hypertensive animals, plus improvement of serum cholesterol profile and triglyceride concentrations, as reviewed recently (Baur and Sinclair 2006; Perez-Vizcaino et al. 2006). Such effects help explain the 'French Paradox' whereby it has been claimed that a moderate red wine consumption could account for the lower rate of cardiovascular disease in the French, whose diet is traditionally high in animal fat (Renaud and de Lorgeril 1992).

The polyphenols in red wine include monomeric flavanols, flavonols, phenolic acids, anthocyanins, proanthocyanins, and stilbene derivates such as resveratrol. Resveratrol (Orallo et al. 2002), together with the anthocyanididin delphnidin (Andriambeloson et al. 1998) and the flavanol quercetin (Flesch et al. 1998), appear to mediate the beneficial physiological effects of red wine polyphenol extracts (RWPE).

The prevention of platelet aggregation by resveratrol involves its selective inactivation of the prostaglandin H_2 synthase, cyclooxygenase (Cox)-1, over Cox-2 (Szewczuk et al. 2004), in much the same way as aspirin exerts its cardioprotective effects. It is also a potent inhibitor of the peroxidase reactions of Cox-1. Its weak inhibition of Cox-2, the isoform targeted by non-steroidal anti-inflammatory drugs, is, moreover, confined to cyclooxygenase activity (Szewczuk et al. 2004). Resveratrol's inhibitory effect is dependent on peroxide substrate and is accompanied by concomitant oxidation of resveratrol at the peroxidase active site. Cox-1 normally synthesizes thromboxane A_2, which is a potent inducer of platelet aggregation and vasoconstriction, whereas inhibition of Cox-2 can increase thrombus formation (Mukherjee et al. 2001).

In addition to its ability to cause vasodilatation by inhibiting thromboxane A_2 formation, resveratrol's vasodilator effect involves stimulation of Ca^{2+}-activated K^+ channels (Li et al. 2000), as well as NO signalling in the endothelium via inhibition of vascular NADH/NADPH oxidase activity, so leading to suppression of superoxide production and thus reduced NO inactivation (Orallo et al. 2002). Resveratrol, but not the other flavonoids, increases expression of genes for eNOS and inducible nitric oxide synthase, iNOS (Leikert et al. 2002; Wallerath et al. 2002; Das et al. 2005; Leighton et al. 2006). Moreover, none of these specific polyphenols affect L-citrulline production by vascular endothelial cells, whereas RWPE do (Leikert et al. 2002). The increase in eNOS in blood vessel walls in response to RWPE and resveratrol contributes to vasodilatation by increasing production of NO (Räthel et al. 2007).

Testing of RWPEs (160 μg/ml) from 180 red wines and a few whites showed marked differences in ability to increase eNOS expression (Räthel et al. 2007). The most potent (6.1-fold increase) was a French Merlot, followed by Syrah and French Pinot noirs (fourfold). White wine extracts had little effect. It appeared that climate, rather than cultivar or growing area determined RWPE potency (Morris 2007; Räthel et al. 2007). The 600 μg/ml of RWPE corresponded to 1–10 μg resveratrol per 750 ml of red wine, i.e., 1–10 μmol/L resveratrol. Even though 10 μM resveratrol significantly increases eNOS promoter, but not enzyme, activity, there is an important contribution from other constituents (Räthel et al. 2007). Perhaps they all work in synergy (Wallerath et al. 2005). Polyphenol extracts of grape *juice* are only slightly less effective, meaning that while vinification increases polyphenol content, it is not necessary for obtaining active extracts (Räthel et al. 2007).

The variation in potency of RWPE from different geographic locations and vintages may have arisen from seasonal and regional variation in climatic conditions. A cold season, for example, could mean higher polyphenol content of the wines that year. This would fit with the xenohormesis hypothesis (Lamming et al. 2004).

There is an association between oxidation of LDL particles and risk of heart disease and myocardial infarction. Resveratrol prevents oxidation of LDL by chelating copper and scavenging ROS (Frankel et al. 1993). Other components of red wine are more effective ROS scavengers, however (Fremont et al. 1999). The fact that resveratrol can be detected in LDL particles after red wine consumption by humans (Urpi-Sarda et al. 2005) is consistent with its ability to prevent peroxidation of lipids and other macromolecules (Baur and Sinclair 2006). Resveratrol can limit cholesterol accumulation by human macrophages by activating transcription factors that target the nuclear liver receptor-α (LXR-α) gene, as well as cholesterol efflux genes *ABCA1* and *ABCG1* which LXR-α influences, and repressing expression of the lipid uptake genes lipoprotein lipase and scavenger receptor SR-AII (Sevov et al. 2006).

Multiple pathways are therefore involved in the beneficial effects of resveratrol and other polyphenols in red wine on cardiovascular health. All of these effects support the inverse association that has been seen between dietary flavonoid consumption and cardiovascular mortality, since the various actions protect against hypertension, ischaemic heart disease, ischaemic damage during myocardial infarction, and brain damage following cerebral ischaemia (Baur and Sinclair 2006; Perez-Vizcaino et al. 2006). In this regard, resveratrol can penetrate the blood-brain barrier to exert strong neuroprotective effects even at low doses of 0.1–1 μg/kg body weight iv (Baur and Sinclair 2006).

Stimulation of Mitochondrial Function and Energy Balance

The enormous potential for resveratrol in human health and disease is highlighted by the recent discovery by David Sinclair's group at Harvard that resveratrol can extinguish most of the ill effects of a high-fat, high-calorie diet in a mouse model of obesity, and risk of diabetes, liver damage and a 30% shorter lifespan, even though the mice stayed fat and had high cholesterol (Baur et al. 2006). This should not be seen as a message to supplement a diet of junk food with resveratrol. When the same dose of resveratrol was given to rats fed a normal diet plasma levels of resveratrol were lower, so these experiments were repeated with a higher dose that gave similar plasma levels as the fat-fed mice. These mice are to complete their lifespans by 2008 and findings will be reported subsequently.

Soon after this study, Johan Auverx' group in France reported in *Cell* that resveratrol, given to mice in high doses, made them resistant to diet-induced obesity and increased their aerobic capacity – muscles burnt more energy, worked more efficiently, and the mice could run twice as far (Lagouge et al. 2006).

Resveratrol activated the sirtuin Sirt1, which, by causing deacetylation, activated peroxisome proliferator-activated receptor γ coactivator (PGC-1), a crucial regulator of mitochondrial biogenesis and function. In muscle this contributes to an increase in oxidative type muscle fibres. As part of this action, each of these studies showed that genes relevant to the changes seen in each tissue were induced, as shown by whole genome expression profiling (Baur et al. 2006; Lagouge et al. 2006). In addition, resveratrol improved insulin sensitivity.

Thus resveratrol, via stimulation of the Sirt1-mediated deacetylation of PGC-1, improves mitochondrial function and energy balance in mice (Baur et al. 2006; Lagouge et al. 2006). In the French study, the mice were young and were fed resveratrol for 3 months to achieve protection from high fat diet-induced obesity (Lagouge et al. 2006). The proportion of slow-twitch/oxidative muscle fibres was increased at the expense of fast-twitch/glycolytic fibres, and genes for oxidative phosphorylation were upregulated, as were mitochondrial genes. This explained why the mice were able to run twice as far before exhaustion (Lagouge et al. 2006). In the US study, the mice fed resveratrol were older, the dose was one tenth as high and they were given resveratrol for a year in order to improve their insulin sensitivity and lifespan when put on a high fat diet (Baur et al. 2006). Despite improved hepatic glucose and lipid metabolism, the mice were not, however, protected from obesity. These mice did not develop hepatic steosis (fatty liver), diabetes, cardiovascular disease or cancer, each of which were seen in the high-fat fed controls. No change in liver histology was observed in the French study, but this could have been contributed by their younger age and the much shorter treatment with resveratrol.

The increase in both studies in deacetylated (thus active) PGC-1α in liver would normally increase gluconeogenesis, but the lowering of glucose observed was attributed to activation by resveratrol of AMP-activated protein kinase (AMPK), which potently inhibits gluconeogenesis. AMPK would also protect from fatty liver, since it increases fatty acid oxidation by inhibiting the rate-limiting enzyme in fatty acid synthesis, acetyl coA carboxylase. AMPK senses changes in stress and energy (low glucose) and may be activated directly by polyphenols (Zang et al. 2006).

The Harvard and French studies published in 2006 highlight a parallel between the Sirt1 and AMPK signalling pathways (Koo and Montminy 2006). Both are triggered by fasting, and are energy sensing in that they respond to changes in NAD^+ and AMP. Each can increase lifespan. They both increase glucose utilization and enhance insulin sensitivity. Each pathway converges on PGC-1α and no doubt other regulators of glucose and lipid metabolism.

A reduction in core body temperature is associated with reduced energy expenditure and improved survival in mice, and *vice versa* (Conti et al. 2006), yet the increased fat metabolism by the mitochondria-rich brown fat leading to more adipose tissue burn off suggests that the higher dose of resveratrol used in the Auverx study was sufficient to trigger Sirt1 activation (Koo and Montminy 2006). The 10–20-fold lower doses of resveratrol in the study by the Sinclair group may explain why core body temperature did not increase in their mice and why their mice were not protected from obesity (Koo and Montminy 2006).

Interestingly, in a case-control study, non-diabetic offspring of Finnish diabetic patients were more likely to show an association of particular alleles of three single nucleotide polymorphisms of the gene, *SIRT1*, with energy expenditure (Lagouge et al. 2006). This offers a possible partial explanation for why different people respond differently to overeating.

Not surprisingly the authors of the French study, as others before them, were tempted to speculate on a role for resveratrol in explaining the French paradox.

Cancer

The initial report that sparked enthusiastic attention towards resveratrol was the discovery that resveratrol given topically to mice reduced skin tumours by 98% (Jang et al. 1997). This led to the finding that initiation and growth of a wide variety of cancers could similarly be prevented by systemically administered resveratrol in rodent models (Baur and Sinclair 2006). Daily doses as low as 200 μg/kg body weight prevented colon cancer in rats (Tessitore et al. 2000). This supports the possibility that dietary sources provide sufficient resveratrol and other polyphenols to have a benefit (Baur and Sinclair 2006). At higher doses (40 mg/kg) 70% of mice survived normally fatal subcutaneous neuroblastomas (Chen et al. 2004). Resveratrol has no effect, however, on breast cancer (Bove et al. 2002). Several phase I clinical trials are underway with up to 7.5 g/day (Baur and Sinclair 2006). Resveratrol reduces risk of various cancers by multiple, complementary mechanisms in experimental models of cancer (Baur and Sinclair 2006). These include reduced activity and gene expression of cyclooxygenases and suppression of ornithine decarboxylase expression (Baur and Sinclair 2006). Each of these enzyme activities are needed for angiogenesis, and 2.5–100 mg/kg resveratrol inhibits tumour-induced neovascularization which is vital for solid tumour growth (Kimura and Okuda 2001; Tseng et al. 2004). It also alters expression of various enzymes, such as cytochrome P450s that are involved in drug metabolism (Baur and Sinclair 2006). Upregulation of Phase II enzymes by resveratrol would reduce carcinogens that may enter the body. A possible down-side might be an alteration in drug pharmacookinetics (Baur and Sinclair 2006). Quinone reductase II is the highest affinity target for resveratrol (Buryanovskyy et al. 2004) and could, by increasing electrophile concentrations, induce expression of Phase II enzymes (Baur and Sinclair 2006). Thus resveratrol may stimulate destruction of carcinogens and at the same time help the body to eliminate harmful molecules (Baur and Sinclair 2006).

As well, resveratrol has anti-profliferative and pro-apoptotic effects (Aggarwal et al. 2004), leading to downregulation of cell cycle proteins and an increase in apoptosis of tumour cells (Baur and Sinclair 2006). Cycling cells exhibit increased susceptibility to resveratrol (Ferry-Dumazet et al. 2002). Resveratrol's action may involve sensitization of tumour cells to other inducers of apoptosis such as tumour necrosis factor-related apoptosis-inducing ligand (TRAIL) (Fulda and Debatin 2004).

Since ROS, by damaging DNA and other macromolecules, can contribute to the initiation and progression of cancer, resveratrol's antioxidant effects could also contribute to its anti-cancer properties (Baur and Sinclair 2006).

Neurological Disorders

Resveratrol confers neuronal protection and offers promise for the treatment and prevention of Alzheimer's disease, Parkinson's disease, Huntington's disease and other neurological disorders (Anekonda 2006). The hallmark of Alzheimer's disease, a progressive age-related, neurodegenerative disorder, is the presence of neurofibrillary tangles and extracellular amyloid beta plaques in the cortex and hippocampus, areas of the brain that are important for memory and learning. Resveratrol activates SIRT1, which, via inhibition of NF-κB signaling, protects against microglia-dependent beta amyloid toxicity (Chen et al. 2005). It also protects neurons from oxidative damage by repressing p53, prevents apoptotic neuronal death and, by suppressing FOXO proteins, promotes neuronal survival (Fig. 5).

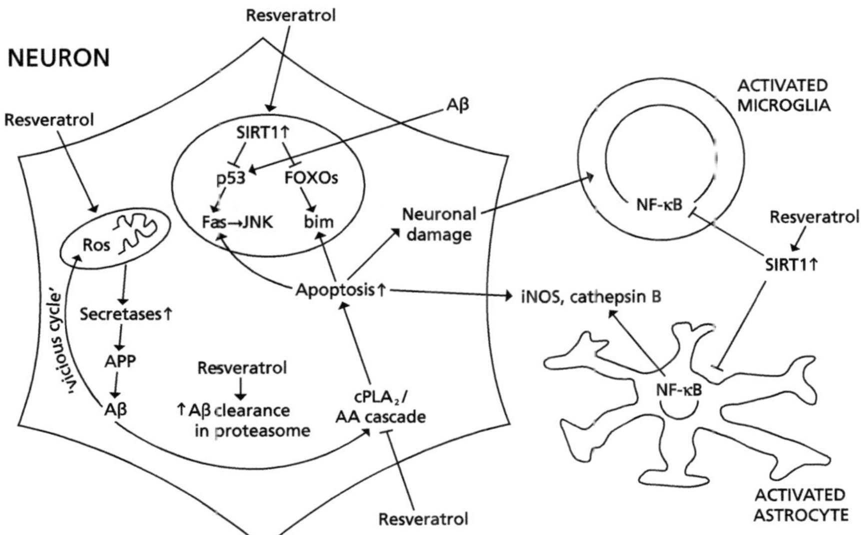

Fig. 5 Neuroprotective mechanisms activated by resveratrol. Abbreviations: AAP, amyloid precursor protein; cPLA2, cytoplasmic phospholipase A_2; FOXOs, forkhead box O transcription factors; iNOS, inducible nitric oxide synthase; NF-κB, nuclear factor κB; SIRT1, sirtun-1 (Modified from Anakonda 2006)

The general cardiovascular protection afforded by resveratrol in the brain is another way in which it protects against Alzheimer's disease. This is because there is some evidence that Alzheimer's is caused by the accumulation of localized neuronal damage surrounding tiny haemorrhagic mini-strokes in the vicinity (Cullen et al. 2006). Resveratrol also protects neurological functions in brain ischaemia, stroke, seizure and epilepsy (Anekonda 2006).

Benefits to Other Organ Systems

Besides its beneficial effects on the heart, blood vessels and brain, resveratrol assists the kidney by not only protecting against carcinogen-induced DNA damage, but also ischaemia reperfusion injury. Such an effect also offers protection in spinal cord trauma, cytokine-induced increased vascular permeability in response to inflammation in liver, as well as harmful effects of toxins on lungs, intestine and colon (see review: (Baur and Sinclair 2006). Resveratrol has, in addition, analgesic effects and can protect against hearing loss.

Ageing

Resveratrol increases the lifespan of all species tested (Table 1). This ability raises the question of whether resveratrol or related compounds might also lengthen human lifespan.

Although resveratrol itself is metabolized rapidly, leading many to doubt that it or its metabolites could have the sorts of beneficial effects seen in earlier *in vitro* studies with high doses, the recent findings in mice lend hope to the possible benefits of new classes of drugs based on resveratrol. As mentioned earlier, polyphenolic compounds, such as resveratrol, mimic the effect of caloric restriction on health and lifespan of the non-human species tested to date. Whereas caloric restriction is challenging for most humans, taking a pill is an easy way to activate similar pathways that should achieve the benefit desired.

Resveratrol and other polyphenols activate similar pathways as calorie restriction (Wood et al. 2004) (Fig. 1). An early target of each of these is the sirtuin class

Table 1 Increase induced by resveratrol in lifespan of various species

Species	Mean (%)	Maximum (%)	Reference
Saccharomyces cerevisiae	70	66	Howitz et al. 2003
Caenorhabditis elegans	18	15	Wood et al. 2004
Drosophila melanogaster	29	22	Bauer et al. 2004; Wood et al. 2004
Nothobranchius furzeri	56	59	Valenzano et al. 2006

of NAD-dependent deacetylases. These activate various pathways such as those shown in Fig. 1. An important action of sirtuins is activation or suppression, depending on cell type and circumstances, of the FOXO group of transcription factors. These then activate specific genes, leading to changes in the cell in levels of certain proteins, may of which are enzymes, resulting in, for example, a decrease in apoptosis, an increase in antioxidant activities, DNA protection, anti-inflammatory effects, and various other mechanisms for promotion of the health of the cell, and thus the organism (reviewed by Morris 2005). A major result of stimulation of pathways controlled by sirtuins may be the enhancement of survival in times of adversity, by ramping up stress resistance pathways in cells (Guarente and Picard 2005). Sirtuins, and indeed the resveratrol-mediated effects, have been conserved through evolution, taking on new roles as new stresses and demands have emerged, which would explain the similar effects they have in diverse species (Koubova and Guarente 2003).

Not surprisingly, overexpression of sirtuins in cultured cells leads to similar effects as resveratrol treatment (Howitz et al. 2003). One effect of resveratrol is to reduce the Michaelis constant (K_m) of Sirt1 by up to 35-fold, and this stimulates p53 deacetylation (Howitz et al. 2003). Suppression of p53 would delay apoptosis, so permitting cells more time to repair damage and prevent needless cell death (Howitz et al. 2003) (Fig. 1). In human HEK 293 cells 0.5 μM resveratrol upregulated *SIRT1* and increased cell survival after exposure to ionizing radiation (Howitz et al. 2003). This involved suppression of Bax-mediated apoptosis (Cohen et al. 2004). Survival and longevity at the cell and organism level appear, moreover, to be intimately linked.

In research conducted in my Laboratory, limited gene expression profiling of human fibroblasts after culture in the presence of resveratrol has identified 47 genes whose expression was altered twofold or more (Stefani et al. 2007). Many were in pathways considered to affect stress-resistance and cell lifespan. Interestingly, two of those suppressed were in the Ras (cancer) pathway (Fig. 6). Resveratrol also suppressed expression of the senescence marker INK4a (recently renamed CDNK2A) (Stefani et al. 2007), that is directly involved in the ageing process (Janzen et al. 2006; Krishnamurthy et al. 2006; Molofsky et al. 2006). Our various results have led us to propose a novel scheme whereby resveratrol's action might, via sirtuins, involve stimulation of the shuttling of cytoplasmic (inactive) FOXOs to the nucleus, where they exert their transcriptional effects to activate stress-resistance and other pathways that, as shown in Fig. 1, assist in cell survival (Stefani et al. 2007).

Dose and Metabolism

Interestingly, Luigi Cornano's diet included 14 oz. of red wine each day. Claims of beneficial effects of resveratrol in animals span a range of 0.1–1,500 mg/kg body weight (Baur and Sinclair 2006). Resveratrol is absorbed rapidly after oral ingestion by humans, but it has a half-life of only 8–14 min, most being converted to sulphate

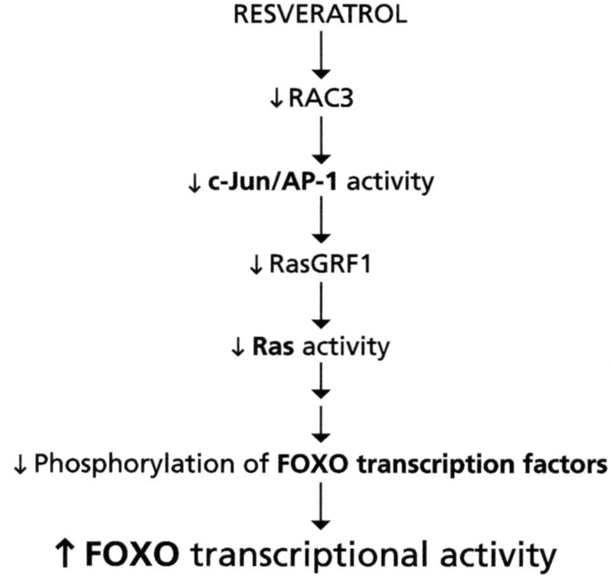

Fig. 6 A possible cancer prevention pathway that may be activated by resveratrol. This represents one of the findings emanating from gene expression profiling experiments in the author's Laboratory in which human dermal fibroblasts were treated with resveratrol, RNA was extracted and was then applied to oligonucleotide arrays to monitor changes in gene expression (Stefani et al. 2007)

conjugates within 30 min (Walle et al. 2004). In contrast, the serum half-life of metabolites of resveratrol is 9.2 h. The levels of resveratrol and its derivatives reached after ingestion of 25 mg in a 70 kg adult are approximately 20–40 nmol/L and 2,000 nmol/L, respectively (Yu et al. 2002). It has been speculated that resveratrol's metabolites might retain or mediate at least some of the beneficial effects (Baur and Sinclair 2006).

The potency of extracts from different grape vine cultivars varies considerably (Räthel et al. 2007). Based on an optimistic estimate of 5 mg/L for the concentration of resveratrol in red wine, two glasses (375 ml) represents a dose of 27 μg/kg in a 70 kg person (Baur and Sinclair 2006). This would result in peak serum concentrations of approximately 2.4 nM of free resveratrol and 180 nM of modified resveratrol. Consumption of 375 ml of red wine daily for 2 weeks results in a plasma polyphenol content of approximately 450 μg/ml (Nigdikar et al. 1998). Although this might be effective in increasing NO in the blood vessel wall (Leikert et al. 2002), so likely providing cardiovascular benefits, it is too low to confer other advantages. Ingestion of a pharmacologically relevant dose of 100 mg/kg/day of resveratrol results in 9 μM authentic resveratrol and 680 μM total resveratrol (Baur and Sinclair 2006). Interestingly, tissues accumulate resveratrol (Vitrac et al. 2003) and resveratrol works in synergy with other dietary compounds (Wallerath et al. 2005). Such interactions might contribute to the beneficial effects of low doses such as in red wine and dietary sources (Baur and Sinclair 2006).

In pure form resveratrol is safe at doses up to 300 mg/kg body weight (Baur and Sinclair 2006). The cost, however, of taking 100 mg/kg body weight per day of a commercial preparation of resveratrol (=7 g/day for a 70 kg person) works out at approximately US $600/month (Baur and Sinclair 2006). Many of the preparations available on the market can, moreover, be substantially depleted of activity by the time they reach the consumer. More stable analogues are, however, being developed.

Alcohol

Although resveratrol has attained notoriety for its health benefits, alcohol itself, at low doses, can confer benefits by lowering cardiovascular risk. The relationship between consumption of ethanol, from any alcoholic beverage, and cardiovascular risk is J-shaped. Moderate intake is associated with a lower risk than no or a higher intake. Thus, by itself, ethyl alcohol could be regarded as a hormetic compound. It should be noted that this applies at the population level only. There is unlikely to be any benefit in someone who has a healthy diet and lifestyle. A major benefit of alcohol may involve its ability to dilate blood vessels. In the liver this leads to increased blood flow and thus uptake of cholesterol for metabolism, so lowering the dangerous forms of cholesterol in people with high cholesterol. Thus overall one would see a population benefit.

The various negative effects of alcohol, however, argue against recommending it. The alcohol component of wine or other beverages can have various detrimental effects, especially as dose rises. Apart from its well-known ability to induce psychomotor impairment increasing the risk of accidents, as well as ethanol's psychosocial effects, both negative and positive, ethanol is mutagenic and carcinogenic. For the latter effect, there is no J-shaped curve – from the lowest doses, alcohol is associated with an ascending risk of cancer (Bagnardi et al. 2001). The World Health Organization has recently reported that five standard drinks per day increases risk of breast cancer by 50%, bowel cancer by 40%, and head and neck cancers by 300%. Breast cancer risk is increased 10% for 1 drink a day, and 43% for 3 drinks a day (30 g alcohol) (Zhang et al. 2007). Moreover, if one were to rely on red wine only as a source of resveratrol (5 mg/L), 100–300 glasses per day would be needed to obtain the daily dose of resveratrol required to confer all of the various health benefits, i.e, the person would succumb to alcohol poisoning first (Baur and Sinclair 2006). One must therefore caution against the use of red wine as a dietary source of resveratrol.

Hormetic Drugs

Such studies as the ones I have discussed in this chapter have fuelled a desire for the use of resveratrol and its more stable synthetic analogs in pharmacotherapy. These compounds would clearly have considerable potential in prevention and treatment of common life-threatening conditions such as type 2 diabetes, cardiovascular disease, cancers and neurodegenerative disorders. By such effects alone, could resveratrol or related compounds lengthen average human lifespan, just as is seen in other species?

Although resveratrol itself is metabolized rapidly, leading many to doubt that it or its metabolites could have the sorts of beneficial effects seen in earlier *in vitro* studies with high doses, the recent findings in mice lend hope to the possibility of new drugs based on resveratrol. Appealingly, as mentioned earlier, polyphenolic compounds like resveratrol mimic the effect of caloric restriction on health and lifespan of the non-human species tested to date. Whereas caloric restriction is challenging for most humans, taking a pill is an easy way to activate similar pathways that might achieve the benefit desired.

From over 35,000 species of vegetables, fruits and nuts one can find more than 4,000 different flavonoids (Howes and Houghton 2003; Howes et al. 2003). Here I have discussed just a few of the most well-known and most extensively tested compounds. There are thousands of published studies, and I have alluded only to a handful of these, hopefully not missing too many of the more important ones. Although the benefits of these various natural chemicals are likely to be similar or overlapping, it will take considerable effort to catalogue them all. The popularity of plant-derived compounds stems from the public perception that being natural they are safer than synthetic drugs, where in the USA, supplements represent a market of over $7 billion/year (Glaser 1999) and exceeds $30 billion worldwide (Raskin et al. 2002).

Conclusions

The remarkable properties of hormetic compounds in helping cells and thus the organism as a whole resist stress can be utilized in a pharmacological sense to help the body prevent or delay the onset of heart disease, stroke, cancer, type 2 diabetes, inflammatory conditions such as arthritis, and neurodegenerative disorders. This will lead to an increase in 'health-span' and thus the average lifespan of the human population. The various polyphenols appear, moreover, to be safe. For example, one needs to consume over 1 g/kg body weight of resveratrol before it registers a toxic effect (Crowell et al. 2004).

The high cost of resveratrol (US $6,800/year for 2.7 kg at a daily dose of 100 mg/kg body weight) has helped provide a motivation for research to develop analogues that are not only cheaper, but that have greater bioavailability, lower metabolism, and also for the discovery of even more effective natural compounds. A potent resveratrol analogue developed by Sirtris Pharmaceuticals, co-founded by David Sinclair at Harvard, has been tested and found to have no adverse effects on healthy men; a clinical trial on diabetes patients is in progress (Check 2006).

The low concentrations of individual flavonoids in food, highlight the needs to derive these compounds from a variety of sources. Stressed plants would seem the obvious source of hormetic compounds. The various flavonoids have, moreover, additive and synergistic effects. Therefore an intake of a combination of flavonoids is most likely going to be preferable to ingestion of one or a few, and consumption of natural sources to get these would appear desirable. The message is thus to increase consumption of polyphenol-rich vegetables, fruit and other sources of these compounds, and heed the other well-known recommendations on what's good for you.

References

Aggarwal BB, Bhardwaj A, Aggarwal RS, Seeram NP, Shishodia S, Takada Y (2004) Role of resveratrol in prevention and therapy of cancer: preclinical and clinical studies (Review). Anticancer Res 24(5A):2783–2840.

Ali RE, Rattan SI (2006) Curcumin's biphasic hormetic response on proteasome activity and heat-shock protein synthesis in human keratinocytes. Ann NY Acad Sci 1067:394–399.

Ambra R, Rimbach G, de Pascual Teresa S, Fuchs D, Wenzel U, Daniel H, Virgili F (2006) Genistein affects the expression of genes involved in blood pressure regulation and angiogenesis in primary human endothelial cells. Nutr Metab Cardiovasc Dis 16:35–43.

Andriambeloson E, Magnier C, Haan-Archipoff G, Lobstein A, Anton R, Beretz A, Stoclet JC, Andriantsitohaina R (1998) Natural dietary polyphenolic compounds cause endothelium-dependent vasorelaxation in rat thoracic aorta. J Nutr 128:2324–2333.

Anekonda TS (2006) Resveratrol – a boon for treating Alzheimer's disease? Brain Res Rev 52:316–326.

Anton S, Melville L, Rena G (2006) Epigallocatechin gallate (EGCG) mimics insulin action on the transcription factor FOXO1a and elicits cellular responses in the presence and absence of insulin. Cell Signal 19:378–383.

Bagnardi V, Blangiardo M, La Vecchia C, Corrao G (2001) A meta-analysis of alcohol drinking and cancer risk. Br J Cancer 85:1700–1705.

Bauer JH, Goupil S, Garber GB, Helfand SL (2004) An accelerated assay for the identification of lifespan-extending interventions in Drosophila melanogaster. Proc Natl Acad Sci USA 101:12980–12985.

Baur JA, Pearson KJ, Price NL, Jamieson HA, Lerin C, Kalra A, Prabhu VV, Allard JS, Lopez-Lluch G, Lewis K, Pistell PJ, Poosala S, Becker KG, Boss O, Gwinn D, Wang M, Ramaswamy S, Fishbein KW, Spencer RG, Lakatta EG, Le Couteur DG, Shaw R, J., Navas P, Puigserver P, Ingram DK, de Cabo R, Sinclair DA (2006) Resveratrol improves health and survival of mice on a high-calorie diet. Nature 444:337–342.

Baur JA, Sinclair DA (2006) Therapeutic potential of resveratrol: the *in vivo* evidence. Nat Rev Drug Discov 5:493–506.

Bloedon LT, Jeffcoat AR, Lopaczynski W, Schell MJ, Black TM, Dix KJ, Thomas BF, Albright C, Busby MG, Crowell JA, Zeisel SH (2002) Safety and pharmacokinetics of purified soy isoflavones: single-dose administration to postmenopausal women. Am J Clin Nutr 76:1126–1137.

Bohm M, Rosenkranz S, Laufs U (2004) Alcohol and red wine: impact on cardiovascular risk (Review). Nephrol Dial Transplant 19:11–16.

Bove K, Lincoln DW, Tsan MF (2002) Effect of resveratrol on growth of 4T1 breast cancer cells in vitro and in vivo. Biochem Biophys Res Commun 291:1001–1005.

Buryanovskyy L, Fu Y, Boyd M, Ma Y, Hsieh TC, Wu JM, Zhang Z (2004) Crystal structure of quinone reductase 2 in complex with resveratrol. Biochemistry 43:11417–11426.

Busby MG, Jeffcoat AR, Bloedon LT, Koch MA, Black T, Dix KJ, Heizer WD, Thomas BF, Hill JM, Crowell JA, Zeisel SH (2002) Clinical characteristics and pharmacokinetics of purified soy isoflavones: single-dose administration to healthy men. Am J Clin Nutr 75:126–136.

Cassidy A (2003) Potential risks and benefits of phytoestrogen-rich diets. Int J Vitam Nutr Res 73:120–126.

Check E (2006) *A votre santé*: now in pill form? Nature 444:11.

Chen J, Zhou Y, Mueller-Steiner S, Chen LF, Kwon H, Yi S, Mucke L, Gan L (2005) SIRT1 protects against microglia-dependent amyloid-beta toxicity through inhibiting NF-kB signaling. J Biol Chem 280:40364–40374.

Chen Y, Tseng SH, Lai HS, Chen WJ (2004) Resveratrol-induced cellular apoptosis and cell cycle arrest in neuroblastoma cells and antitumor effects on neuroblastoma in mice. Surgery 136:57–66.

Chen YM, Ho SC, Lam SS, Ho SS, Woo JL (2003) Soy isoflavones have a favorable effect on bone loss in Chinese postmenopausal women with lower bone mass: a double-blind, randomized, controlled trial. J Clin Endocrinol Metab 88:4740–4747.

Christen Y (2004) *Ginko biloba* and neurodegenerative disorders. Frontiers Biosci 9:3091–3104.

Christen Y, Maixent J-M (2002) What is *Ginko biloba* extract Egb 761? An overview – from molecular biology to clinical medicine. Cell Mol Biol 48:601–611.

Cohen HY, Miller C, Bitterman KJ, Wall NR, Hekking B, Kessler B, Howitz KT, Gorospe M, de Cabo R, Sinclair DA (2004) Calorie restriction promotes mammalian cell survival by inducing the SIRT1 deacetylase. Science 305:390–392.

Conti B, Sanchez-Alavez M, Winsky-Sommerer R, Morale MC, Lucero J, Brownell S, Fabre V, Huitron-Resendiz S, Henriksen S, Zorrilla EP, de Lecea L, Bartfai T (2006) Transgenic mice with a reduced core body temperature have an increased life span. Science 314:825828.

Crowell JA, Korytko PJ, Morrissey RL, Booth TD, Levine BS (2004) Resveratrol-associated renal toxicity. Toxicol Sci 82:614–619.

Cullen KM, Kócsi Z, Stone J (2006) Microvascular pathology in the aging human brain: evidence that senile plaques are sites of microhaemorrhages. Neurobiol Aging 27:1786–1796.

Das S, Alagappan VK, Bagchi D, Sharma HS, Maulik N, Das DK (2005) Coordinated induction of iNOS-VEGF-KDR-eNOS after resveratrol consumption: a potential mechanism for resveratrol preconditioning of the heart. Vascul Pharmacol 42:281–289.

Ehrnhoefer DE, Duennwald M, Markovic P, Wacker JL, Engemann S, Roark M, Legleiter J, Marsh JL, Thompson LM, Lindquist S, Muchowski PJ, Wanker EE (2006) Green tea (-)-epigallocatechin-gallate modulates early events in huntingtin misfolding and reduces toxicity in Huntington's disease models. Hum Mol Genet 15:2743–2751.

Everitt AV (2003) Food restriction, pituitary hormones and ageing. Biogerontology 4:47–50.

Fang MZ, Wang Y, Ai N, Hou Z, Sun Y, Lu H, Welsh W, Yang CS (2003) Tea polyphenol (-)-epigallocatechin-3-gallate inhibits DNA methyltransferase and reactivates methylation-silenced genes in cancer cell lines. Cancer Res 63:7563–7570.

Ferry-Dumazet H, Garnier O, Mamani-Matsuda M, Vercauteren J, Belloc F, Billiard C, Dupouy M, Thiolat D, Kolb JP, Marit G, Reiffers J, Mossalayi MD (2002) Resveratrol inhibits the growth and induces the apoptosis of both normal and leukemic hematopoietic cells. Carcinogenesis 23:1327–1333.

Fisher ND, Hughes M, Gerhard-Herman M, Hollenberg NK (2003) Flavanol-rich cocoa induces nitric-oxide-dependent vasodilation in healthy humans. J Hypertens 21:2281–2286.

Flesch M, Schwarz A, Bohm M (1998) Effects of red and white wine on endothelium-dependent vasorelaxation of rat aorta and human coronary arteries. Am J Physiol 275:H1183–H1189.

Fontana L, Meyer TE, Klein S, Holloszy JO (2004) Long-term calorie restriction is highly effective in reducing the risk for atherosclerosis in humans. Proc Natl Acad Sci USA 101:6659–6663.

Frankel EN, Waterhouse AL, Kinsella JE (1993) Inhibition of human LDL oxidation by resveratrol. Lancet 341:1103–1104.

Fremont L, Belguendouz L, Delpal S (1999) Antioxidant activity of resveratrol and alcohol-free wine polyphenols related to LDL oxidation and polyunsaturated fatty acids. Life Sci 64:2511–2521.

Fujiki H (2005) Green tea: health benefits as cancer preventive for humans. Chem Rec 5:119–132.

Fulda S, Debatin KM (2004) Sensitization for tumor necrosis factor-related apoptosis-inducing ligand-induced apoptosis by the chemopreventive agent resveratrol. Cancer Res 64:337–346.
Glaser V (1999) Billion-dollar market blossoms as botanicals take root. Nat Biotechnol 17:17–18.
Green NS, Foss TR, Kelly JW (2005) Genistein, a natural product from soy, is a potent inhibitor of transthyretin amyloidosis. Proc Natl Acad Sci USA 102:14545–14550.
Grinberg LN, Newmark H, Kitrossky N, Rahamim E, Chevion M, Rachmilewitz EA (1997) Protective effects of tea polyphenols against oxidative damage to red blood cells. Biochem Pharmacol 54:973–978.
Guarente L, Kenyon C (2000) Genetic pathways that regulate ageing in model organisms. Nature 408:255–262.
Guarente L, Picard F (2005) Calorie restriction – the SIR2 connection. Cell 120:473–482.
Guo Q, Zhao B, Li M, Shen S, Xin W (1996) Studies on protective mechanisms of four components of green tea polyphenols against lipid peroxidation in synaptosomes. Biochim Biophys Acta 1304:210–212.
Guo Q, Zhao B, Shen S, Hou J, Hu J, Xin W (1999) ESR study on the structure-antioxidant activity relationship of tea catechins and their epimers. Biochim Biophys Acta 1427:13–23.
Hider RC, Liu ZD, Khodr HH (2001) Metal chelation of polyphenols. Methods Enzymol 335:190–203.
Higdon JV, Frei B (2003) Tea catechins and polyphenols: health effects, metabolism, and antioxidant functions. Crit Rev Food Sci Nutr 43:89–143.
Hodgson JM (2006) Effects of tea and tea flavonoids on endothelial function and blood pressure: a brief review. Clin Exp Pharmacol Physiol 33:838–841.
Hollenberg NK (2006) Vascular action of cocoa flavanols in humans: the roots of the story. J Cardiovasc Pharmacol 47(Suppl. 2):S99–S102.
Houston MC (2005) Nutraceuticals, vitamins, antioxidants, and minerals in the prevention and treatment of hypertension. Prog Cardiovasc Dis 47:396–449.
Howes MJ, Houghton PJ (2003) Plants used in Chinese and Indian traditional medicine for improvement of memory and cognitive function. Pharmacol Biochem Behav 75:513–527.
Howes MJ, Perry NS, Houghton PJ (2003) Plants with traditional uses and activities, relevant to the management of Alzheimer's disease and other cognitive disorders. Phytother Res 17:1–18.
Howitz KT, Bitterman KJ, Cohen HY, Lamming DW, Lavu S, Wood JG, Zipkin RE, Chung P, Kisielewski A, Zhang LL, Scherer B, Sinclair DA (2003) Small molecule activators of sirtuins extend *Saccharomyces cerevisiae* lifespan. Nature 425:191–196.
Jang M, Cai L, Udeani GO, Slowing KV, Thomas CF, Beecher CW, Fong HH, Farnsworth NR, Kinghorn AD, Mehta RG, Moon RC, Pezzuto JM (1997) Cancer chemopreventive activity of resveratrol, a natural product derived from grapes. Science 275:218–220.
Janzen V, Forkert R, Fleming HE, Saito Y, Waring MT, Dombkowski DM, Cheng TH, DePinho RA, Sharpless NE, Scadden D (2006) Stem-cell ageing modified by the cyclin-dependent kinase inhibitor $p16^{INK4a}$. Nature 443:421–426.
Jiang F, Dusting GJ (2003) Natural phenolic compounds as cardiovascular therapeutics: potential role of their antiinflammatory effects. Curr Vasc Pharmacol 1:135–156.
Kaliora AC, Dedoussis GV, Schmidt H (2006) Dietary antioxidants in preventing atherogenesis (Review). Atherosclerosis 187:1–17.
Kao YH, Hiipakka RA, Liao S (2000) Modulation of endocrine systems and food intake by green tea epigallocatechin gallate. Endocrinology 141:980–987.
Kimura Y, Okuda H (2001) Resveratrol isolated from *Polygonum cuspidatum* root prevents tumor growth and metastasis to lung and tumor-induced neovascularization in Lewis lung carcinoma-bearing mice. J Nutr 131:1844–1849.
Koo S-H, Montminy M (2006) In vino veritas: a tale of two Sirt1s? Cell 127:1091–1093.
Koubova J, Guarente L (2003) How does calorie restriction work? Genes Dev 17:313–321.
Krishnamurthy J, Ramsey MR, Ligon KL, Torrice C, Koh A, Bonner-Weir S, Sharpless NE (2006) $p16^{INK4a}$ induces an age-dependent decline in islet regenerative potential. Nature 443:453–457.

Kuzuhara T, Sei Y, Yamaguchi K, Suganuma M, Fujiki H (2006) DNA and RNA as new binding targets of green tea catechins. J Biol Chem 281:17446–17456.

Lagouge M, Argmann C, Gerhart-Hines Z, Meziane H, Lerin C, Daussin F, Messadeq N, Milne J, Lambert P, Elliott P, Geny B, Laakso M, Puigserver P, Auwerx J (2006) Resveratrol Improves mitochondrial function and protects against metabolic disease by activating SIRT1 and PGC-1a. Cell 127:1109–1122.

Lambert JD, Yang CS (2003) Mechanisms of cancer prevention by tea constituents. J Nutr 133:3262S–3267S.

Lamming DW, Wood JG, Sinclair DA (2004) Small molecules that regulate lifespan: evidence for xenohormesis (Review). Mol Microbiol 53:1003–1009.

Le Bourg E, Minois N (2005) Does dietary restriction really increase longevity in *Drosophila melanogaster*? Ageing Res Rev 4:409–421.

Le Bourg E, Rattan SIS (2006) Can dietary restriction increase longevity in all species, particularly in human beings? Introduction to a debate among experts. Biogerontology 7:123–125.

Leighton F, Miranda-Rottmann S, Urquiaga I (2006) A central role of eNOS in the protective effect of wine against metabolic syndrome. Cell Biochem Funct 24:291–298.

Leikert JF, Rathel TR, Wohlfart P, Cheynier V, Vollmar AM, Dirsch VM (2002) Red wine polyphenols enhance endothelial nitric oxide synthase expression and subsequent nitric oxide release from endothelial cells. Circulation 106:1614–1617.

Li C, Allen A, Kwagh J, Doliba NM, Qin W, Najafi H, Collins HW, Matschinsky FM, Stanley CA, Smith TJ (2006) Green tea polyphenols modulate insulin secretion by inhibiting glutamate dehydrogenase. J Biol Chem 281:10214–10221.

Li HF, Chen SA, Wu SN (2000) Evidence for the stimulatory effect of resveratrol on Ca^{2+} -activated K^{+} current in vascular endothelial cells. Cardiovasc Res 45:1035–1045.

Loh KP, Low LS, Wong WH, Zhou S, Huang SH, De Silva R, Duan W, Chou WH, Zhu YZ (2006) A comparison study of cerebral protection using Ginkgo biloba extract and Losartan on stroked rats. Neurosci Lett 398:28–33.

Mandel SA, Avramovich-Tirosh Y, Reznichenko L, Zheng H, Weinreb O, Amit T, Youdim MB (2005) Multifunctional activities of green tea catechins in neuroprotection. Modulation of cell survival genes, iron-dependent oxidative stress and PKC signaling pathway. Neurosignals 14:46–60.

McCay CM, Crowell MF, Maynard LA (1935) The effect of retarded growth upon the length of life span and upon the ultimate body size. 1935. Nutrition 5:155–171.

McCullough ML, Chevaux K, Jackson L, Preston M, Martinez G, Schmitz HH, Coletti C, Campos H, Hollenberg NK (2006) Hypertension, the Kuna, and the epidemiology of flavanols. J Cardiovasc Pharmacol 47(Suppl. 2):S103–S109.

Molofsky AV, Slutsky SG, Joseph NM, He S, Pardal R, Krishnamurthy J, Sharpless NE, Morrison SJ (2006) Increasing $p16^{INK4a}$ expression decreases forebrain progenitors and neurogenesis during ageing. Nature 443:448–452.

Morris BJ (2005) A forkhead in the road to longevity: the molecular basis of lifespan becomes clearer (Review). J Hypertens 23:1285–1309.

Morris BJ (2007) Climate not cultivars in the NO-ing of red wines. J Hypertens 25:501–503.

Mukherjee D, Nissen SE, Topol EJ (2001) Risk of cardiovascular events associated with selective COX-2 inhibitors. JAMA 286:954–959.

Nigdikar SV, Williams NR, Griffin BA, Howard AN (1998) Consumption of red wine polyphenols reduces the susceptibility of low-density lipoproteins to oxidation *in vivo*. Am J Clin Nutr 68:258–265.

Orallo F, Alvarez E, Camina M, Leiro JM, Gomez E, Fernandez P (2002) The possible implication of *trans*-resveratrol in the cardioprotective effects of long-term moderate wine consumption. Mol Pharmacol 61:294–302.

Park OJ, Surh YJ (2004) Chemopreventive potential of epigallocatechin gallate and genistein: evidence from epidemiological and laboratory studies. Toxicol Lett 150:43–56.

Peng G, Dixon DA, Muga SJ, Smith TJ, Wargovich MJ (2006) Green tea polyphenol (-)-epigallocatechin-3-gallate inhibits cyclooxygenase-2 expression in colon carcinogenesis. Mol Carcinog 45:309–319.

Perez-Vizcaino F, Duarte J, Andriantsitohaina R (2006) Endothelial function and cardiovascular disease: effects of quercetin and wine polyphenols (Review). Free Radic Res 40:1054–1065.
Perona JS, Cabello-Moruno R, Ruiz-Gutierrez V (2006) The role of virgin olive oil components in the modulation of endothelial function (Review). J Nutr Biochem 17:429–445.
Raskin I, Ribnicky DM, Komarnytsky S, Ilic N, Poulev A, Borisjuk N, Brinker A, Moreno DA, Ripoll C, Yakoby N, O'Neal JM, Cornwell T, Pastor I, Fridlender B (2002) Plants and human health in the twenty-first century. Trends Biotechnol 20:522–531.
Räthel TR, Samtleben R, Vollmar AM, Dirsch VM (2007) Activation of endothelial nitric oxide synthase by red wine polyphemols: impact of grape cultivars, growing area and the vinification process. J Hypertens 25:541–549.
Ravindranath MH, Muthugounder S, Presser N, Viswanathan S (2004) Anticancer therapeutic potential of soy isoflavone, genistein. Adv Exp Med Biol 546:121–165.
Renaud S, de Lorgeril M (1992) Wine, alcohol, platelets, and the French paradox for coronary heart disease. Lancet 339:1523–1526.
Rivas M, Garay RP, Escanero JF, Cia P, Jr., Cia P, Alda JO (2002) Soy milk lowers blood pressure in men and women with mild to moderate essential hypertension. J Nutr 132:1900–1902.
Sánchez M, Galisteo M, Vera R, Villar IC, Zarzuelo A, Tamargo J, Perez-Vizcaino F, Duarte J (2006) Quercetin downregulates NADPH oxidase, increases eNOS activity and prevents endothelial dysfunction in spontaneously hypertensive rats. J Hypertens 24:75–84.
Sarkar FH, Li Y (2002) Mechanisms of cancer chemoprevention by soy isoflavone genistein. (Review). Cancer Metastasis Rev 21:265–280.
Sevov M, Elfineh L, Cavelier LB (2006) Resveratrol regulates the expression of LXR-alpha in human macrophages. Biochem Biophys Res Commun 348:1047–1054.
Smith JV, Burdick AJ, Golik P, Khan I, Wallace D, Luo Y (2002) Anti-apoptotic properties of Ginkgo biloba extract EGb 761 in differentiated PC12 cells. Cell Mol Biol (Noisy-le-grand) 48:699–707.
Stefani M, Markus MA, Lin RCY, Pinese M, Dawes IA, Morris BJ (2007) The effect on resveratrol on a cell model of human aging. Ann NY Acad Sci (in press).
Szewczuk LM, Forti L, Stivala LA, Penning TM (2004) Resveratrol is a peroxidase-mediated inactivator of COX-1 but not COX-2: a mechanistic approach to the design of COX-1 selective agents. J Biol Chem 279:22727–22737.
Tessitore L, Davit A, Sarotto I, Caderni G (2000) Resveratrol depresses the growth of colorectal aberrant crypt foci by affecting bax and $p21^{CIP}$ expression. Carcinogenesis 16:1619–1622.
Tseng SH, Lin SM, Chen JC, Su YH, Huang HY, Chen CK, Lin PY, Chen Y (2004) Resveratrol suppresses the angiogenesis and tumor growth of gliomas in rats. Clin Cancer Res 10:2190–2202.
Turner R (2003) Tuned for longer life. Nature 423:125.
Urpi-Sarda M, Jauregui O, Lamuela-Raventos RM, Jaeger W, Miksits M, Covas MI, Andres-Lacueva C (2005) Uptake of diet resveratrol into the human low-density lipoprotein. Identification and quantification of resveratrol metabolites by liquid chromatography coupled with tandem mass spectrometry. Anal Chem 77:3149–3155.
Valenzano DR, Terzibasi E, Genade T, Cattaneo A, Domenici L, Cellerino A (2006) Resveratrol prolongs lifespan and retards the onset of age-related markers in a short-lived vertebrate. Curr Biol 16:296–300.
Visioli F, Galli C (1994) Oleuropein protects low density lipoprotein from oxidation. Life Sci 55:1965–1971.
Vitrac X, Desmouliere A, Brouillaud B, Krisa S, Deffieux G, Barthe N, Rosenbaum J, Merillon JM (2003) Distribution of [^{14}C]-trans-resveratrol, a cancer chemopreventive polyphenol, in mouse tissues after oral administration. Life Sci 72:2219–2233.
Walford RL, Mock D, Verdery R, MacCallum T (2002) Calorie restriction in Biosphere 2: alterations in physiological, haematological, and biochemical parameters in humans restricted for a 2-year period. J Gerontol 57A:B211–B224.
Walle T, Hsieh F, DeLegge MH, Oatis JE, Jr., Walle UK (2004) High absorption but very low bioavailability of oral resveratrol in humans. Drug Metab Dispos 32:1377–1382.

Wallerath T, Deckert G, Ternes T, Anderson H, Li H, Witte K, Forstermann U (2002) Resveratrol, a polyphenolic phytoalexin present in red wine, enhances expression and activity of endothelial nitric oxide synthase. Circulation 106:1652–1658.

Wallerath T, Li H, Godtel-Ambrust U, Schwarz PM, Forstermann U (2005) A blend of polyphenolic compounds explains the stimulatory effect of red wine on human endothelial NO synthase. Nitric Oxide 12:97–104.

Wang ZY, Huang MT, Lou YR, Xie JG, Reuhl KR, Newmark HL, Ho CT, Yang CS, Conney AH (1994) Inhibitory effects of black tea, green tea, decaffeinated black tea, and decaffeinated green tea on ultraviolet B light-induced skin carcinogenesis in 7,12-dimethylbenz[a]anthracene-initiated SKH-1 mice. Cancer Res 54:3428–3435.

Wood JG, Rogina B, Lavu S, Howitz K, Helfand SL, Tatar M, Sinclair D (2004) Sirtuin activators mimic caloric restriction and delay ageing in metazoans. Nature 430:686–689.

Yu C, Shin YG, Chow A, Li Y, Kosmeder JW, Lee YS, Hirschelman WH, Pezzuto JM, Mehta RG, van Breemen RB (2002) Human, rat, and mouse metabolism of resveratrol. Pharm Res 19:1907–1914.

Zang M, Xu S, Maitland-Toolan KA, Zuccollo A, Hou X, Jiang B, Wierzbicki M, Verbeuren TJ, Cohen RA (2006) Polyphenols stimulate AMP-activated protein kinase, lower lipids, and inhibit accelerated atherosclerosis in diabetic LDL receptor-deficient mice. Diabetes 55:2180–2191.

Zhang SM, Lee IM, Manson JE, Cook NR, Willett WC, Buring JE (2007) Alcohol consumption and breast cancer risk in the Women's Health Study. Am J Epidemiol 165:667–676.

Zimmermann M, Colciaghi F, Cattabeni F, Di Luca M (2002) *Ginko biloba* extract: from molecular mechanisms to the treatment of Alzheimer's disease. Cell Mol Biol 48:613–623.

Chapter 9
Mild Stress in the Aging Heart

Role of Ischemic Preconditioning

Pasquale Abete[1] and Franco Rengo[2]

Introduction

Hormetic effects have been documented in diverse combinations of stressors and recipient organism. Such sublethal stress pre-treatments have been shown to increase stress resistance and life expectancy in several animal organisms. Stressors reported to increase subsequent stress resistance include heat, cold, hypergravity, and pesticides. Increased life span has been reported after a similarly diverse number of hormetic treatments including heat, cold, hypergravity, ionizing radiation, exercise, electric shock, and wounding accompanied by regrowth (Martinez 1996; Minois 2000). Khazaeli et al. (1997) have demonstrated that heat induced longevity extension in *Drosophila* and, similarly, Michalski et al. increased longevity in *Caenorhabditis elegans* by heating stress (2001). Resistance to the paradoxical effects of hormesis necessitated the extended and exhaustive documentation of the phenomenon, an effort led primarily by Edward Calabrese (Kaiser 2003). Those efforts produced both practical and theoretical benefits. The practical benefit was an additional set of tools useful in studying survival, following the application of mild stress. The theoretical aspect was further support for the inverse correlation observed between stress resistance generally and improved survival.

The biological mechanisms underlying hormesis are unclear. Transcription, translation, and/or post-translational protein medication, such as phosphorylation may represent the hormetic response. Calabrese and Baldwin (1986) have suggested

[1]Cattedra di Geriatria – Dipartimento di Medicina Clinica, Scienze Cardiovascolari ed Immunologiche, University of Naples "Federico II", Italy.

[2]Cattedra di Geriatria – Dipartimento di Medicina Clinica, Scienze Cardiovascolari ed Immunologiche, University of Naples; "Federico II"; Scientific Director, Istituto Scientifico di Telese Terme, Fondazione Salvatore Maugeri, IRCCS, Benevento, Italy.

Address for correspondence:
Pasquale Abete, M.D., Ph.D., Dipartimento di Medicina Clinica e Scienze Cardiovascolari ed Immunologiche, Cattedra di Geriatria, Università degli Studi di Napoli "Federico II", Via S. Pansini, 5, 80131 Napoli, Italy. Tel: +39-081-7462270;
Fax: +39-081-7462339; e-mail: p.abete@unina.it

E. Le Bourg and S.I.S. Rattan (eds.), *Mild Stress and Healthy Aging.*

that "*… no single hormetic mechanism is expected, but a common evolutionary-based homeostasis maintenance regulatory strategy is evident*". These authors underline that a hormetic response may reflect either a direct stimulation or an overcompensation response. Minois (2000) has proposed that hormesis is a consequence of metabolic regulation coupled to the expression of stress response proteins. These two hypotheses are not reciprocally exclusive and they may represent a multiple pathway for a single mechanism.

Hormetic Effect of Ischemic Preconditioning

Ischemic preconditioning is an adaptive mechanism in response to brief episodes of myocardial ischemia able to reduce the cellular damage subsequent to a more prolonged ischemic damage; in other words, a brief period of ischemia and the following reperfusion makes the heart more resistant to successive more prolonged ischemic insult, and therefore ischemic preconditioning is able to reduce the infarct size (Murry et al. 1986). Cardiac ischemic preconditioning, the most powerful endogenous protective mechanism, is represented as an anti-ischemic vaccination. In other words, ischemic preconditioning is a classical example of a hormetic effect of a mild stress (i.e., brief and multiple ischemic episodes) able to get a protection in the heart against the more prolonged ischemic insult (Kloner et al. 1998; Napoli et al. 2000; Yellon et al. 2003).

This mechanism does not depend on collateral vessels: ischemic preconditioning is present in animal models without collateral vessel and in experimental model as in the isolated perfused heart subjected to a global ischemia (Kloner et al. 1998; Napoli et al. 2000; Yellon et al. 2003). The protective effect of ischemic preconditioning could be reduced if the time between preconditioning ischemic episode and the prolonged ischemic episode is excessive. Finally, ischemic preconditioning is classified in "early" when the protective effect is manifest immediately after an ischemic episode and "delayed" when the protective effect is manifest 24 h from ischemic episodes (Kloner et al. 1998; Napoli et al. 2000; Yellon et al. 2003).

Several studies have demonstrated that adenosine and/or norepinephrine and/or endogenous opioids may be the trigger of ischemic preconditioning at the molecular level (Kloner et al. 1998; Napoli et al. 2000; Yellon et al. 2003). One possibility is the α_{1b}-adrenergic (Banerjee et al. 1993; Hu and Nattel 1995) stimulation by norepinephrine by means of G-protein inhibitory activation (G_i), sensible to pertussin, with a transient increment of C phospholipase activity and, consequently, of diacylglycerol with the activation of protein kinase C (Fig. 1). This protein, in its different isoforms, is associated to different receptors and physiological effects (Mitchell et al. 1995). The δ-isoform, translocated into cell membrane seems to be responsible of the "early" protective mechanism throughout K-channel ATP-dependent mechanism at mitochondrial level while the ε-isoform, translocated at the nuclear level, seems to be responsible of the "delayed" protective mechanism throughout the synthesis of the "heat shock proteins" (Kloner et al. 1998; Napoli et al. 2000; Yellon et al. 2003).

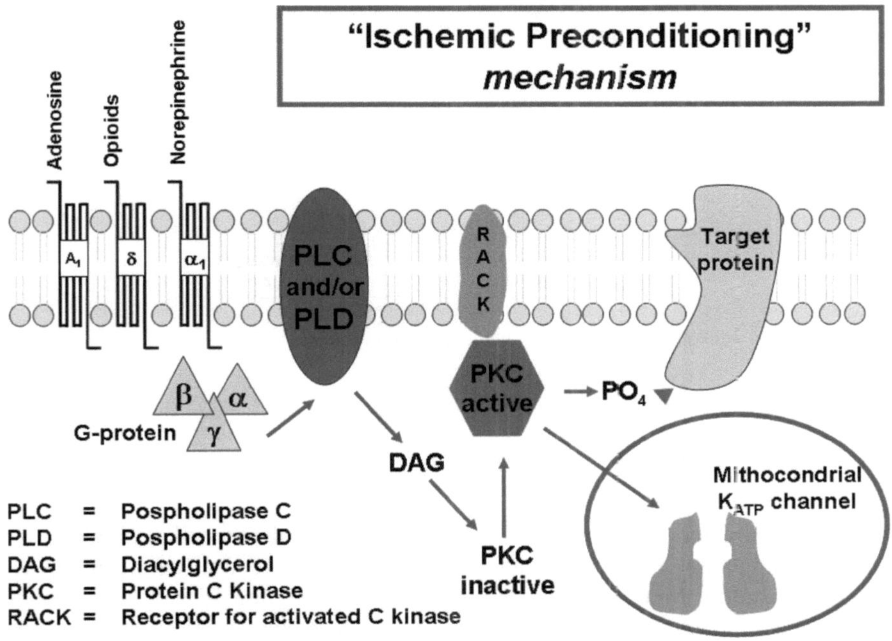

Fig. 1 The hypothetical mechanism of ischemic preconditioning (see the text for details)

Clinical Evidences of Ischemic Preconditioning

Clinical observations of ischemic preconditioning are very important because if the mechanism were elucidated, it should become the basis of a new therapeutical approach of coronary artery diseases. Clinical equivalents of ischemic preconditioning are represented by transluminaly coronary angioplasty, preinfarction angina, walk through angina and warm-up phenomenon (Kloner et al. 1998; Napoli et al. 2000; Yellon et al. 2003). In particular, Kloner et al. (1995) show that in patients with preinfarction angina at least 48 h before myocardial infarction, the incidence of mortality and cardiogenic shock was reduced. Successively, Andreotti et al. (1996) have demonstrated that patients with preinfarction angina who underwent thrombolytic therapy showed a more rapid reperfusion, and a reduction of infarct size. Finally, three phenomena of clinical relevance should be considered in which the mechanism seems to be the ischemic preconditioning: the first one is represented by a condition of effort angina following physical exercise, which paradoxically disappears when the exercise keeps on going ("walk-through angina"); the second one is characterized by a reduction of clinical and electrocardiographic parameters of effort ischemia following the first exercise test ("Warm-up phenomenon"); the last one is represented by transluminal coronary angioplasty: electrocardiographic, biochemical and clinical signs of ischemia are reduced after the first balloon inflation (Kloner et al. 1998; Napoli et al. 2000; Yellon et al. 2003) (Fig. 2).

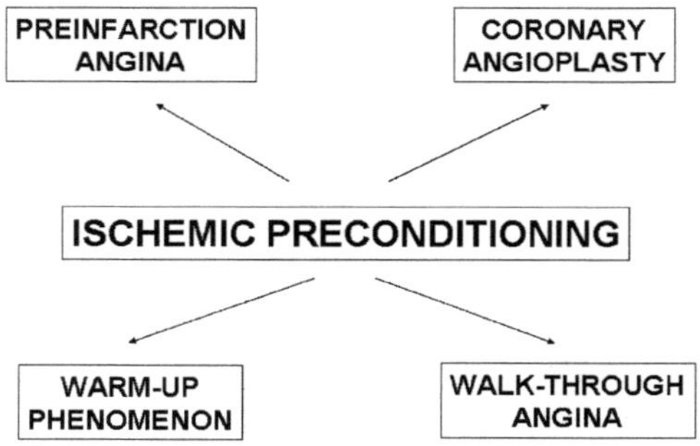

Fig. 2 Clinical equivalents of cardiac ischemic preconditioning

Age-Dependent Reduction of Ischemic Preconditioning

Several investigators have supported the idea that ischemic preconditioning may be reduced with aging. Why? Age is a powerful predictor of mortality for acute myocardial infarction. Mortality for acute myocardial infarction is 80% in coronary heart disease patients older than 65 years, with a frequency threefold greater compared with adult patients (Weaver et al. 1991; Gurwitz et al. 1996; Tresch et al. 1996; Berger et al. 2000; Boersma et al. 2000; Napoli et al. 2002; Maggioni et al. 1993). These characteristics have been attributed to several conditions such as myocardial mass increase (Gerstenblith et al. 1977), diastolic relaxation (Tresch and McGough 1995) and reduced angiogenesis (Rivard et al. 1999). Although the high rate of comorbidity and the reduction of thrombolytic therapy observed in the elderly seem to be the more reasonable explanations (Berger et al. 2000; Boersma et al. 2000; Napoli et al 2002; Tofler et al. 1988), no factor completely explains the age-related increase of acute myocardial infarction mortality. Thus, the higher mortality and morbidity associated with advancing age could be due to the reduction of some endogenous protective mechanism against myocardial ischemia, a classic example being "ischemic preconditioning".

Experimental studies have demonstrated that myocardial ischemia may determine a greatest myocardial dysfunction in heart from senescent animals with a less evident recovery during reperfusion when compared to adult ones (Ataka et al. 1992; Abete et al. 1995; Abete et al. 1999). From these evidences stems the hypothesis that anti-ischemic endogenous mechanisms such as ischemic preconditioning may reduce with aging. Thus, we have firstly demonstrated, in the isolated and perfused rat heart, that ischemic preconditioning is reduced in hearts from rats 24 months old that underwent 20 min of ischemia and 40 min of reperfusion and in rats subjected to a preconditioning protocol with a short period of ischemia (2 min) followed by 10 min of reperfusion. The results obtained showed an improvement of left ventricular function in hearts from adult but not in those from senescent rats (Fig. 3A). In addition, norepinephrine release from coronary effluent was reduced in senescent

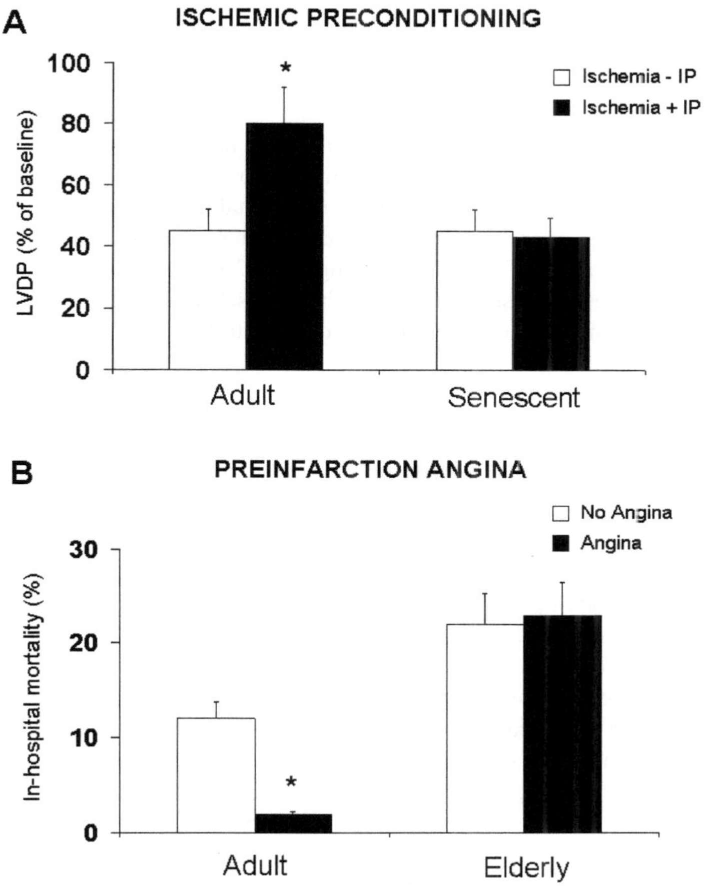

Fig. 3 The age-related reduction of ischemic preconditioning in the isolated and perfused rat heart is shown in (**A**): bar graphs show percentage recovery value at the end of reperfusion of left ventricular developed pressure (LVDP): in adult and in senescent hearts subjected to ischemia for 20 min and reperfused for 40 min (Ischemia – IP); in adult and in senescent hearts treated with preconditioning transient ischemic stimulus for 2 min followed by 10 min of reperfusion and then a standard ischemia-reperfusion insult (ischemic perfusion for 20 min and reperfused for 40 min) (Ischemia + IP) (*$p < 0.01$ vs Ischemia – IP). The age-related reduction of preinfarction angina, a clinical equivalent of ischemic preconditioning, is shown in (**B**): bar graphs show percentage recovery value of in-hospital mortality of adult and elderly patients without and with preinfarction angina (*$p < 0.01$ vs No Angina)

hearts in response to preconditioning stimulus when compared to adult ones. In adult animals the pre-treatment with reserpine was able to deplete norepinephrine from adrenergic store and the recovery of left ventricular function during reperfusion was abolished. The study allowed to conclude that ischemic preconditioning is reduced with aging and this reduction is due to a reduction of norepinephrine release in response to preconditioning stimulus (Abete et al. 1996). Moreover, the age-related reduction of ischemic preconditioning has been successively confirmed in several studies. Tani et al. (1997) demonstrated that hearts became more vulnerable to ischemia with age and that the beneficial effects of preconditioning were reversed in middle-aged rat hearts. Ischemic preconditioning reduced necrosis development and enhanced reperfusion contractile function in young but not in aged hearts (Fenton et al. 2000). Moreover, not only ischemic stimulus but also pharmacological means such as adenosine A1 agonist, protein kinase C analog, and mitochondrial ATP-sensitive potassium channel opener diazoxide are unable to precondition the aging heart (Schulman et al. 2001). Finally, Bartling et al. (2003) have shown that ischemic preconditioning has no positive effect on the postischemic functional recovery of senescent human myocardium in human right atrial trabeculae.

Clinical Evidence of the Age-Related Reduction of Ischemic Preconditioning: The Preinfarction Angina

Preinfarction angina, the most evident equivalent of ischemic preconditioning, has been studied in adult and elderly patients in terms of in-hospital primary and secondary events: in adult patients (<65 years), both in-hospital mortality and cardiogenic shock were more frequent in the absence than in the presence of preinfarction angina; CK-MB (creatine kinase myoglobin fraction) peak, transmural infarctions number, the incidence of ventricular tachycardia and fibrillation, and the ventricular dysfunction were significantly higher in the adult patients without than in those with preinfarction angina (Fig. 3B). In elderly patients (≥65 years), the protective effect of preinfarction angina seems to be lost: both in-hospital primary (mortality and cardiogenic shock) and secondary (CK-MB peak, transmural infarctions number, the incidence of ventricular tachycardia and fibrillation, and the ventricular dysfunction) end-points were similar in elderly patients with and without preinfarction angina (Fig. 3B). Logistic regression, adjusted for several variables including the use of thrombolytic and anti-anginal therapy, demonstrated that preinfarction angina is a protective variable against mortality and cardiogenic shock in adult but not in elderly patients (Abete et al. 1997). Successively, in non-elderly patients, prodromal angina was associated with lower peak creatine kinase levels, lower in-hospital mortality rates, and better 5-year survival rates while in elderly patients there was no significant difference in peak creatine kinase levels, in-hospital mortality rate, and 5-year survival rates. A multivariate analysis showed that prodromal angina in the 24 h before infarction was associated with 5-year survival rate in non-elderly patients but not in elderly patients (Ishihara et al. 2000). The "warm-up phenomenon" also seems to reduce in elderly patients as demonstrated both with dynamic electrocardiography (Napoli et al. 1999) and effort exercise (Longobardi et al. 2000): with both methods the ischemic episode successive to the first myocardial ischemia was reduced in adult but not in elderly patients. Very recently, the absence of ischemic preconditioning has been demonstrated in elderly patients during coronary angioplasty (Lee et al. 2002).

Thus, ischemic preconditioning seems to represent a classical example of hormesis which is reduced with aging. Why the most powerful protective mechanism against ischemia is lost with aging? Mild stresses such as brief ischemic episodes are able to get the adult but not the senescent heart more resistant to prolonged myocardial ischemia.

One hypothesis is that mild stress, and therefore ischemic preconditioning, is operative only when the aging is accompanied by corrected lifestyles. Dietary restriction increases the resistance of organisms to stress and has been shown to activate stress resistance pathways in cells in different tissues. Another example of an environmental factor that may improve health by a hormesis-based mechanism is exercise, which is well-known to inflict oxidative and metabolic stress on the musculoskeletal and cardiovascular systems (Radak et al. 2005).

Caloric Restriction and Exercise Training in the Aging Heart

Caloric restriction has been widely described as an anti-aging intervention (Masoro 2000; Starnes and Rumsey 1988; Yu 1999). In particular, caloric restriction increases the life span of rodents (McCay et al. 1935), retards the severity of some age-related diseases (Weindruch and Walford 1988) and attenuates the physiological decline of several organs, including the heart (Masoro 2000; Yu 1999; Klebanof et al. 1997). Specifically, caloric restriction enhances arterial baroreflexes (Cavagnini and Mancia 1998), isoproterenol sensitivity (Herlihy 1984) and prevents the age-related impairments in diastolic function (Taffet et al. 1997). Recently, we have demonstrated that ischemic preconditioning improved both mechanical and electrical parameters in adult but not in hearts from ad libitum fed senescent animals and that ischemic preconditioning is preserved in food-restricted senescent animals. In addition, caloric restriction seems to restore ischemic preconditioning in hearts from senescent animals through an involvement of the adrenergic pathway in response to ischemic preconditioning. Norepinephrine release in response to ischemic preconditioning is reduced in the senescent heart and restored in hearts from food-restricted senescent animals (Abete et al. 2002) (Fig. 4A).

Exercise training is able to increase average survival time in rats without increasing their maximal longevity (Holloszy 1997) but it might reverse several age-related modification of the heart. More specifically, exercise training antagonizes the age-related prolongation of isometric contraction, action potential duration (Li et al. 1986), age-related decrease of Ca-ATPase of the sarcoplasmic reticulum (Tate et al. 1986), adenylate cyclase depression and G_{1a} increase (Bohm et al. 1993), and attenuates age-associated diastolic dysfunction in rats (Brenner et al. 2001). The effects on mechanical parameters of ischemic preconditioning against 20 min of global ischemia followed by 40 min of reperfusion has been investigated in isolated perfused hearts from adult (6 months) and sedentary or trained (6 weeks of graduated swim training) senescent (24 months) rats. The effect of preconditioning on developed pressure recovery was absent in sedentary but present in trained senescent

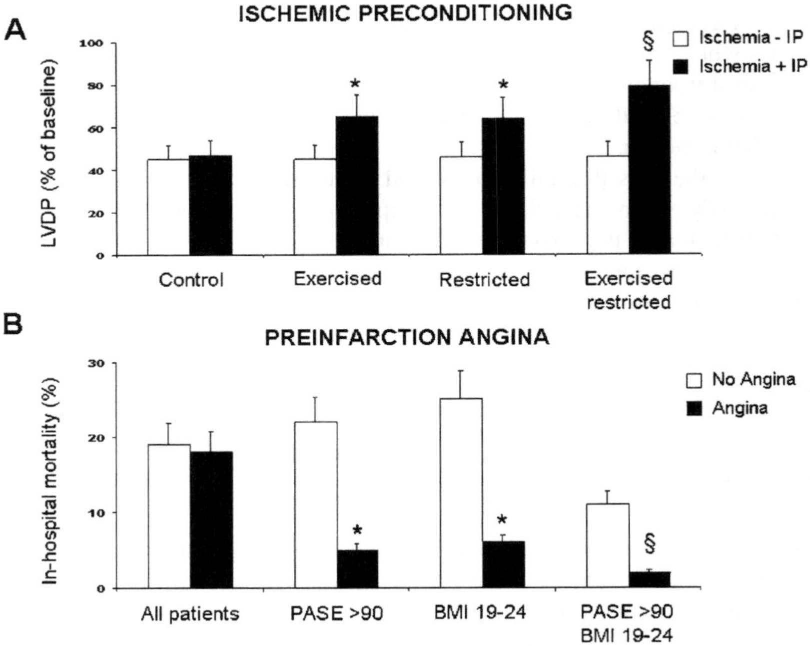

Fig. 4 Restoring of the age-related of ischemic preconditioning by exercise training and caloric restriction in the isolated and perfused rat heart is shown in (**A**): bar graphs show showing percentage recovery value at the end of reperfusion of left ventricular developed pressure (LVDP) in sedentary ad libitum fed (control), trained ad libitum fed, sedentary food-restricted and trained- and food-restricted senescent hearts. The heart was subjected to ischemia for 20 min and reperfused for 40 min (Ischemia - IP) and treated with preconditioning transient ischemic stimulus for 2 min followed by 10 min of reperfusion and then a standard ischemia-reperfusion insult (ischemic perfusion for 20 min and reperfused for 40 min) (Ischemia + IP) (* $p < 0.01$ vs Control Ischemia – IP; §$p < 0.01$ vs exercised and trained Ischemia + IP). Preserving of the age-related reduction of preinfarction angina, clinical equivalent of ischemic preconditioning, by physical activity and normal BMI is shown in (**B**): bar graphs show percentage recovery value of in-hospital mortality of adult and elderly patients without and with preinfarction angina (*$p < 0.01$ vs all patients; §$p < 0.05$ vs PASE > 90 and BMI = 19–24)

hearts (Fig. 4A). Norepinephrine release significantly increased after preconditioning in adult and in trained but not in sedentary senescent hearts. Thus, in adult and trained but not in sedentary senescent hearts, preconditioning reduces postischemic dysfunction and is associated with an increase in norepinephrine release (Abete et al. 2000).

"Combined action" of physical activity and caloric restriction can retard the age-related modifications of the heart. In isoproterenol-induced acute myocardial infarction in male rats both exercise or maintenance of body weight are able separately to prevent drug-induced acute myocardial infarction, but additional protection is produced when food restriction is combined with exercise training (Crandall et al. 1981). Combined exercise and food restriction is able to decrease fatigue in the gastrocnemius muscle and to improve muscle bioenergetics (Horska et al. 1999). Since ischemic preconditioning may be partially corrected by exercise training and food restriction the role of exercise training combined with food restriction on restoring ischemic preconditioning was investigated in isolated hearts (Abete et al. 2005). Developed pressure recovery was partial in hearts from trained ad libitum fed and sedentary food-restricted but it was total in adult hearts and in those from trained and food restricted senescent rats (Fig. 4A). Thus, the combined action of exercise training and food restriction is able to completely restore the ischemic preconditioning in the aging heart. In these experimental conditions, cardiac norepinephrine release in response to ischemic preconditioning stimulus is reduced in senescent but not in adult animals and is partially restored by exercise training and by dietary restriction in senescent animals. Interestingly, cardiac norepinephrine release in response to ischemic preconditioning stimulus is completely restored in trained and food-restricted animals, demonstrating that the synergistic action on norepinephrine release might explain how exercise training and food restriction together are able to totally preserve ischemic preconditioning in the aging heart. This hypothesis was supported by the complete abolition of the restoring effect of exercise training and food restriction after reserpine pre-treatment which is able to deplete norepinephrine stores (Abete et al. 2005).

Ischemic Preconditioning and Norepinephrine Release

In the rat experimental model, one of the possible mechanisms of ischemic preconditioning is the release of norepinephrine in response to ischemic preconditioning stimulus by α_1-adrenoreceptor stimulation (Banerjee et al. 1993; Hu et al. 1995). The abolition of ischemic preconditioning mechanism by prazosin and reserpine strongly suggests that the endogenous release of catecholamines mediates the effect of ischemic preconditioning. The age-related decline of tissue catecholamines due to several mechanisms, including a related diminished ability for catecholamine synthesis (Mazzeo and Horvarth 1987; Dawson and Meldrum, 1992), could explain the reduction of preconditioning in the aging heart.

It has been demonstrated that anti-aging interventions such as exercise training and caloric restriction are able to restore norepinephrine release from cardiac adrenergic terminations in response to stress stimulus (Mazzeo et al. 1987; Raisin et al. 1983; Kim et al. 1994). Accordingly, it has been recently showed that exercise training re-establishes ischemic preconditioning in trained senescent rats through an increase of norepinephrine in response to an ischemic preconditioning stimulus (Abete et al. 2000). Caloric restriction affects adrenergic system in several ways. First of all, caloric restriction is accompanied by a reduction in plasma norepinephrine (Raisin et al 1983). In addition, it has also been demonstrated that the norepinephrine content of hearts from food-restricted rats was higher than controls; in addition, the cardiac synaptosomal P_2 fraction from food-restricted rats possessed higher norepinephrine content than the P_2 fraction of ad libitum fed control rats

(Kim et al. 1994). Interestingly, Snyder et al. (1998) demonstrated that aging reduces the capacity of cardiac adrenergic nerve terminals to release norepinephrine and this age-related reduction is significantly blunted by dietary restriction. Similarly, cardiac norepinephrine release in response to ischemic preconditioning stimulus is more reduced in senescent than in adult animals. However, cardiac norepinephrine release in response to preconditioning stimulus is restored in food-restricted senescent animals. This finding might be one of the mechanisms by which dietary restriction restores ischemic preconditioning in the aging heart. The absence of ischemic preconditioning in adult and food-restricted senescent animals with depleted norepinephrine stores by reserpine confirms this hypothesis (Abete et al. 2002).

It is reasonable to suppose that a hormetic response such as ischemic preconditioning may be mediated by a norepinephrine release, which is expected to occur after a mild stress. It is convincing that the age-related norepinephrine release reduction may be restored by anti-aging interventions such as exercise training and caloric restriction and to be again available to trigger the ischemic preconditioning.

Effects of Physical Activity and Hypocaloric Diet on Reducing Morbidity and Mortality in the Elderly

Several epidemiological studies indicate that physical activity offers partial protection against primary or secondary events of cardiovascular diseases and associated mortality among middle-aged and older men (Hu et al. 2004). In the Goteborg study, the most active men, after 20 years of follow-up, had a relative risk of death from coronary heart disease of 0.72 (Rosengren and Wilhelmsen 1997). In the British Regional Heart Study, light, moderate and vigorous activity reduced mortality and heart attacks in older men by 0.61, 0.50, 0.65, respectively. In the Honolulu Heart Program, the risk of coronary heart disease was reduced in physically capable elderly men with the distance walked (Wannamethee et al. 1998). In this study, men who walked <0.25 mile/day had a twofold increased risk of coronary heart disease versus those who walked >1.5 mile/day, and more importantly, men who walked 0.25–1.5 mile/day were also at a significantly higher risk of coronary heart disease than men who walked longer distances (Hakim et al. 1999). These findings suggest that the risk of coronary heart disease is reduced in physically capable elderly men. Several factors are involved in this positive effect of physical activity: a lipid-lowering effect (Weintraub et al. 1989), increased insulin sensitivity (Wannamethee et al. 2000), reduced arterial pressure (Engstrom et al. 1999), increased coronary vasodilatory capacity and coronary perfusion (Haskell et al. 1993), correction of endothelial dysfunction (Hambrecht et al. 2000), the anti-arrhythmic effect due to the reduction of heart rate and sympathetic activity (Palatini 1999), and coronary vasorelaxation depending on nitric oxide bioavailability (Linke et al. 2006).

The correlation between body–mass index, cardiovascular mortality and age is very intricate. The influence of being overweight or obese on hospital mortality was studied in patients with acute myocardial infarction. When stratified according to age, 30% of obese patients ≥65 years died in the hospital compared to 6% of obese patients <65 years: the multivariate analysis showed that obesity was an independent predictor of death at the hospital in the older, but not in the younger patient subset (Hoit et al. 1987). Successively, Stevens et al. (1998) reported that an increased body–mass index was associated with an increased cardiovascular mortality, but the phenomenon progressively declined with aging. In fact, a unit BMI increase was related to an increase of cardiovascular mortality risk of 1.10 between 30 and 44 years but it decreased to 1.03 in patients aged between 65 and 74 years. Finally, Calle et al. (1999) have demonstrated that a high body–mass index is related to an increased cardiovascular mortality risk in all age groups including subjects older than 75 years. In this case, the relative risk of mortality increased from 2.30 in subjects aged 30–64 years to 2.75 in subjects aged 65–74 years old, but it decreased to 1.53 in subjects older than 75 years. However, the absolute risk increased progressively from 659 deaths/100,000 in subjects aged 30–64 years to 6154 deaths/100,000 in subjects older than 75 years (Calle et al. 1999). Overweight is associated with hypercholesterolemia (Ettinger et al. 1992), hyperinsulinemia (Chisholm et al. 1997), hypertriglyceridemia (Jeppesen et al. 1998) and increased plasminogen activator inhibitor activity (Vague et al. 1986), all predictive factors for the development of coronary heart disease in elderly obese patients.

Few studies are performed on determining the benefits of the combined action of physical activity and body–mass index in the elderly. Recently, in a Longitudinal study in the Healthy Ageing (HALE), comprising 1,507 men and 332 apparently healthy women, aged 70–90 years enrolled in the "Survey in Europe on Nutrition and the Elderly a Concerned Action" (SENECA) and the "Finland, Italy, the Netherlands, Elderly" (FINE), the single and combined effect of Mediterranean diet, being physically active, moderate alcohol use, and non-smoking on ten-year mortality from all causes, coronary heart disease, cardiovascular diseases, and cancer were studied (Knoops et al. 2004). Physical activity, non-smoking, Mediterranean diet, and moderate alcohol use reduced the risk of cardiovascular disease mortality. More importantly, the combination of 2, 3 and 4 low-risk patterns lowered progressively the mortality risk for cardiovascular disease. Moreover, a lack of adherence to this low-risk pattern was associated with a population attributable risk of 61% from cardiovascular diseases (Knoops et al. 2004). Recently, a study of 18,892 Finnish men and women aged 25–74 years without history of coronary heart disease, stroke, or heart failure at baseline has been published. Physical activity, different indicators of obesity, education, smoking, blood pressure, total and high-density lipoprotein cholesterol and history of diabetes were measured at baseline. An incident cardiovascular disease event was defined as the first stroke or coronary heart disease event or cardiovascular disease death based on national hospital discharge and mortality register data. Physical inactivity and the obesity indicators both predicted cardiovascular disease risk in men, but in women the joint effect was inconsistent (Hu et al. 2004). Few data about the mechanisms on the combined action of physical activity and body–mass index on coronary heart disease in the elderly are available. Katzel et al. (1997) reported the effects of physical activity and weight loss on cardiac risk factors in older men. Physical activity and weight loss had a more substantial impact than physical activity alone on glucose tolerance and lipoprotein concentrations. It has been also demonstrated that aerobic exercise and weight loss are effective in lowering blood pressure and improving glucose metabolism, but the combined action determines a further improvement in glucose metabolism (Dengel et al. 1998).

It is widely accepted that lifestyle interventions should prevent cardiovascular disease by reducing some of the classic cardiovascular risks. However, all these conditions are not sufficient to explain the beneficial effect of lifestyle interventions in the elderly: a classical example is the hypercholesterolemia, frequently associated to physical inactivity and obesity, which is known to decrease with age (Ettinger et al. 1992). So, what happens in the elderly? One hypothesis should be that both lifestyle interventions stimulate hormetic response and restore and/or preserve some endogenous protective mechanism, which is known to reduce with aging, i.e., "ischemic preconditioning".

Effects of Physical Activity and Hypocaloric Diet on Preinfarction Angina, a Clinical Equivalent of Ischemic Preconditioning, in the Elderly

The effects of physical activity, evaluated by the PASE (Physical Activity Scale for the Elderly) (Washburn et al. 1999), on preinfarction angina, a clinical equivalent of ischemic preconditioning, was investigated in adult and elderly patients with acute myocardial infarction. A high level of physical activity was strongly associated with reduced in-hospital mortality. Moreover, a high level of physical activity reduced in-hospital mortality in elderly patients with but not in those without preinfarction angina (Fig. 4B). Accordingly, regression analysis confirmed that the protective effect of preinfarction angina is preserved in elderly patients with a high level of physical activity (Abete et al. 2001).

Accordingly, less in-hospital deaths were observed in elderly patients with than in those without preinfarction angina in the subset of patients with the lowest body–mass index (Fig. 4B). Regression analysis demonstrated that preinfarction angina did not protect against in-hospital death when analyzed in all patients independently of body–mass index, whereas it was protective in the subset of patients with the lowest body–mass index (Abete et al. 2003).

Preliminary data evaluating the mortality for acute myocardial infarction in elderly subjects stratified both for physical activity and body–mass index indicate that acute myocardial infarction-related mortality decreases with increasing physical activity and decreasing body–mass index. This phenomenon is absent in elderly patients without preinfarction angina but is particularly evident in elderly patients with preinfarction angina (Fig. 4B). The synergistic action of physical activity and low body–mass index is confirmed by the multivariate analysis of preinfarction angina on in-hospital death performed by stratifying for PASE quartiles combined with each body–mass index quartile. Preinfarction angina was protective against in-hospital death in the highest PASE score in all body–mass index subgroups. Interestingly, preinfarction angina reached the maximum at highest PASE and lowest body–mass index score and it was still protective against in-hospital death at 57–90 PASE score but at lowest body–mass index. More importantly, the effect of preinfarction angina is "predictive" of mortality in sedentary and overweight elderly patients, but it becomes "protective" in trained normal weight elderly patients, suggesting a key role of lifestyles in this phenomenon.

Conclusions

We conclude that:

1. Hormesis in the heart is a complex mechanism by which the heart is immunized from pathological insults such as myocardial ischemia.
2. A mild stress such as brief ischemic episodes may protect the heart from a successive and more prolonged myocardial ischemia (ischemic preconditioning).
3. This mechanism is reduced with aging and it may be restored and/or preserved by lifestyle interventions such as physical activity and/or hypocaloric diet.

These emerging findings suggest that many of the environmental factors that improve health and survival by reducing cardiovascular morbidity and mortality (for example, dietary restriction and exercise training) may exert their beneficial effects through a hormesis-like mechanism.

References

Abete P, Cioppa A, Ferrara P, Caccese P, Ferrara N, Rengo F (1995) Reduced aerobic metabolic efficiency in postischemic myocardium dysfunction in rats: role of aging. Gerontology 41:187–194.

Abete P, Ferrara N, Cioppa A, Ferrara P, Bianco S, Calabrese C, Cacciatore F, Longobardi G, Rengo F (1996) Preconditioning does not prevent post-ischemic dysfunction in aging heart. J Am Coll Cardiol 27:1777–1786.

Abete P, Ferrara N, Cacciatore F, Madrid A, Bianco S, Calabrese C, Napoli C, Scognamiglio P, Bollella O, Cioppa A, Longobardi G, Rengo F (1997) Angina-induced protection against myocardial infarction in adult and senescent patients. A loss of preconditioning mechanism in aging heart. J Am Coll Cardiol 30:947–954.

Abete P, Cioppa A, Calabrese C, Pascucci I, Cacciatore F, Napoli C, Carnovale V, Ferrara N, Rengo F (1999) Ischemic threshold and myocardial stunning in the aging heart. Exp Geront 34:875–884.

Abete P, Calabrese C, Ferrara N, Cioppa A, Pisanelli P, Cacciatore F, Longobardi G, Napoli C, Rengo F (2000) Exercise training restores ischemic preconditioning in the aging heart. J Am Coll Cardiol 36:643–650.

Abete P, Ferrara N, Cacciatore F, Sagnelli E, Manzi M, Carnovale V, Calabrese C, de Santis D, Testa G, Longobardi G, Napoli C, Rengo F (2001) High level of physical activity preserves the

cardioprotective effect of preinfarction angina in elderly patients. J Am Coll Cardiol 38:1357–1365.
Abete P, Testa G, Ferrara N, De Santis D, Capaccio P, Viati L, Calabrese C, Cacciatore F, Longobardi G, Condorelli M, Napoli C, Rengo F (2002) Cardioprotective effect of ischemic preconditioning is preserved in food-restricted senescent rats. Am J Physiol 282: H1978–H1987.
Abete P, Cacciatore F, Ferrara N, Calabrese C, de Santis D, Testa G, Galizia G, Del Vecchio S, Leosco D, Condorelli M, Napoli C, Rengo F (2003) Body mass index and preinfarction angina in elderly patients with acute myocardial infarction. Am J Clin Nutr 78:796–801.
Abete P, Testa G, Galizia G, Mazzella F, Della Morte D, de Santis D, Calabrese C, Cacciatore F, Gargiulo G, Ferrara N, Rengo G, Sica V, Napoli C, Rengo F (2005) Tandem action of exercise training and food restriction completely preserves ischemic preconditioning in the aging heart. Exp Gerontol 40:43–50.
Andreotti F, Pasceri V, Hackett DR, Davies GJ, Haider AW, Maseri A (1996) Preinfarction angina as a predictor of more rapid coronary thrombolysis in patients with acute myocardial infarction. N Engl J Med 334:7–12.
Ataka K, Chen D, Levitsky S, Jimenez E, Feinberg H (1992) Effect of aging on intracellular Ca^{2+}, pH_i, and contractility during ischemia and reperfusion. Circulation 86(II):371–376.
Banerjee A, Locke-Winter C, Rogers KB, Mitchell MB, Brew EC, Cairns CB, Bensard DD, Harken AH (1993) Preconditioning against myocardial dysfunction after ischemia and reperfusion by an α1-adrenergic mechanism. Circ Res 73:656–670.
Bartling B, Friedrich I, Silber RE, Simm A (2003) Ischemic preconditioning is not cardioprotective in senescent human myocardium. Ann Thorac Surg 76:105–111.
Berger AK, Radford MJ, Wang Y, Krumholz HM (2000) Thrombolytic therapy in older patients. J Am Coll Cardiol 36:366–374.
Boersma E, Pieper KS, Steyerberg EW, Wilcox RG, Chang WC, Lee KL, Akkerhuis KM, Harrington RA, Deckers JW, Armstrong PW, Lincoff AM, Califf RM, Topol EJ, Simoons ML (2000) Predictors of outcome in patients with acute coronary syndromes without persistent ST-segment elevation. Results from an international trial of 9461 patients. The PURSUIT Investigators. Circulation 101:2557–2567.
Bohm M, Dorner H, Htun P, Lensche H, Platt D, Erdmann E (1993) Effects of exercise on myocardial adenylate cyclase and Gi alpha expression in senescence. Am J Physiol 264:H805–H814.
Brenner DA, Apstein CS, Saupe KW (2001) Exercise training attenuates age-associated diastolic dysfunction in rats. Circulation 104:221–226.
Calabrese EJ and Baldwin LA (1986) Defining hormesis. Hum Exp Toxicol 21:91–97.
Calle EE, Thun MJ, Petrelli JM, Rodriguez C, Heath CW Jr (1999) Body-mass index and mortality in a prospective cohort of US Adult. N Engl J Med 15:1097–1105.
Cavagnini F, Mancia G (1998) Body weight reduction, sympathetic nerve traffic, and arterial baroreflex in obese normothensive humans. Circulation 97:2037–2042.
Chisholm DJ, Campbell LV, Kraegen EW (1997) Pathogenesis of the insulin resistance syndrome (syndrome X). Clin Exp Pharmacol Physiol 24:782–784.
Crandall DL, Feirer RP, Griffith DR (1981) Relative role of caloric restriction and exercise training upon susceptibility to isoproterenol-induced myocardial infarction in male rats. Am J Clin Nutr 34:841–847.
Dawson R, Meldrum MJ (1992) Norepinephrine content in cardiovascular tissue from the aged Fisher 344 rat. Gerontology 38:185–191.
Dengel DR, Galecki AT, Hagberg JM, Pratley RE (1998) The independent and combined effects of weight loss and aerobic exercise on blood pressure and oral glucose tolerance in older men. Am J Hypertens 11:1405–1412.
Engstrom G, Hedblad B, Janzon L (1999) Hypertensive men who exercise regularly have lower rate of cardiovascular mortality. J Hypertens 17:737–742.
Ettinger WH, Wahl PW, Kuller LH, Bush TL, Tracy RP, Manolio TA, Borhani NO, Wong ND, O'Leary DH (1992) Lipoprotein lipids in older people. Results from the Cardiovascular Health Study. The CHS Collaborative Research Group. Circulation 86:858–869.

Fenton RA, Dickson EW, Meyer TE, Dobson JG Jr (2000) Aging reduces the cardioprotective effect of ischemic preconditioning in the rat heart. J Mol Cell Cardiol 32:1371–1375.

Gerstenblith G, Frederiksen J, Yin FC, Fortuin NJ, Lakatta EG, Weisfeldt ML (1977) Echocardiography assessment of a normal adult aging population. Circulation 56:672–679.

Gurwitz JH, Gore JM, Goldberg RJ, Rubison M, Chandra N, Rogers WJ (1996) Recent age-related trends in the use of thrombolytic therapy on patients who have had acute myocardial infarction. Ann Intern Med 124:283–291.

Hakim AA, Curb JD, Petrovitch H, Rodriguez BL, Yano K, Ross GW, White LR, Abbott RD (1999) Effects of walking on coronary heart disease in elderly men: the Honolulu Heart Program. Circulation 100:9–13.

Hambrecht R, Wolf A, Gielen S, Linke A, Hofer J, Erbs S, Schoene N, Schuler G (2000) Effect of exercise on coronary endothelial function in patients with coronary artery disease. N Engl J Med 342:454–460.

Haskell WL, Sims C, Myll J, Bortz WM, St Goar FG, Alderman EL (1993) Coronary artery size and dilating capacity in ultra-distance runners. Circulation 87:1076–1082.

Herlihy JT (1984) Dietary manipulation of cardiac and aortic smooth muscle reactivity to isoproterenol. Am J Physiol 246:H369–H373.

Hoit BD, Gilpin EA, Maisel AA (1987) Influence of obesity on morbidity and mortality after acute myocardial infarction. Am Heart J 114:1334–1341.

Holloszy JO (1997) Mortality rate and longevity of food-restricted exercising male rats: a re-evaluation. J Appl Physiol 82:399–403.

Horska A, Brant LJ, Ingram DK, Hansford RG, Roth GS, Spencer RG (1999) Effect of long-term caloric restriction and exercise on muscle bioenergetics and force development in rats. Am J Physiol 276:E766–E773.

Hu G, Tuomilehto J, Silventoinen K, Barengo N, Jousilahti P (2004) Joint effects of physical activity, body mass index, waist circumference and waist-to-hip ratio with the risk of cardiovascular disease among middle-aged Finnish men and women. Eur Heart J 25:2212–2219.

Hu K, Nattel S (1995) Mechanisms of ischemic preconditioning in rat hearts. Involvement of α_{1b}-adrenoreceptors, pertussin toxin-sensitive G proteins, and protein kinase C. Circulation 92:2259–2265.

Ishihara M, Sato H, Tateishi H, Kawagoe T, Shimatani Y, Ueda K, Noma K, Yumoto A, Nishioka K (2000) Beneficial effect of prodromal angina pectoris is lost in elderly patients with acute myocardial infarction. Am Heart J 139:881–888.

Jeppesen J, Hein HO, Suadicani P, Gyntelberg F (1998) Triglyceride concentration and ischemic heart disease. An eight-year follow-up in the Copenaghen Male Study. Circulation 97:1029–1036.

Kaiser J (2003) Sipping from a poisoned chalice. Science 302:376–379.

Katzel LI, Bleecker ER, Rogus EM, Goldberg AP (1997) Sequential effects of aerobic exercise training and weight loss on risk factors for coronary disease in healthy, obese middle-aged and older men. Metabolism 46:1441–1447.

Khazaeli AA, Tatar M, Pletcher SD, Curtsinger JW (1997) Heat induced longevity extension in Drosophila I. Heat treatment, mortality, and Thermotolerance. J Gerontol 52A:B48–B52.

Kim SW, Yu BP, Sander M (1994) Dietary restriction modulates the norepinephrine content and uptake of the heart and cardiac synaptosomal. Proc Soc Exp Boil Med 207:43–47.

Klebanov S, Herlihy JT, Freemna GL (1997) Effect of long-term food restriction on cardiac mechanics. Am J Physiol 273:H2333-H2342.

Kloner RA, Shook T, Przyklenk K, Davis VG, Junio L, Matthews RV, Burstein S, Gibson M, Poole WK, Cannon CP (1995) Previous angina alters in-hospital outcome in TIMI 4: a clinical correlate to preconditioning. Circulation 91:37–47.

Kloner RA, Bolli R, Marban E, Reinlib L, Braunwald E (1998) Medical and cellular implications of stunning, hibernation and preconditioning. An NHLBI workshop. Circulation 97:1848–1867.

Knoops KT, de Groot LC, Kromhout D, Perrin AE, Moreiras-Varela O, Menotti A, van Staveren WA (2004) Mediterranean diet, lifestyle factors, and 10-year mortality in elderly European men and women: the HALE project. JAMA 292:1433–1439.

Lee TM, Su SF, Chou TF, Lee YT, Tsai CH (2002) Loss of preconditioning by attenuated activation of myocardial ATP-sensitive potassium channel in elderly patients undergoing coronary angioplasty. Circulation 105:334–340.

Li Y, Lincoln T, Mendelowitz D, Grossman W, Wei JY (1986) Age-related differences in effect of exercise training on cardiac muscle function in rats. Am J Physiol 251:H12–H18.

Linke A, Erbs S, Hambrecht R (2006) Exercise and the coronary circulation-alterations and adaptations in coronary artery disease. Prog Cardiovasc Dis 48:270–284.

Longobardi G, Abete P, Ferrara N, Papa A, Rosiello R, Furgi G, Calabrese C, Cacciatore F, Rengo F (2000) Warm-up. Phenomenon in adult and elderly patients with coronary artery disease. Further evidence of the loss of.ischemic preconditioning. in the aging heart. J Gerontol 55: M124–M129.

Maggioni AP, Maseri A, Fresco C, Franzosi MG, Mauri F, Santoro E, Tognoni G (1993) Age related increase in mortality among patients with first myocardial infarctions treated with thrombolysis. N Engl J Med 329:1442–1448.

Martinez DE (1996) Rejuvenation of the disposable soma: repeated injury extends lifespan in an asexual annelid. Exp Gerontol 31:699–704.

Masoro EJ (2000) Caloric restriction and aging: an update. Exp Gerontol 35:299–305.

Mazzeo RS, Colburn RW, Horvath SM (1987) Effect of aging and endurance training on tissue catecholamine response to strenuous exercise in Fischer 344 rats. Metabolism 35:602–607.

Mazzeo RS, Horvarth SM (1987) A decline in myocardial and hepatic norepinephrine turnover with age in Fisher 344 rats. Am J Physiol 252:E762–E764.

McCay CM, Crowell MF, Maynard LA (1935) The effect of retarded growth upon the length of life span and upon the ultimate body size. J Nutr 10:63–79.

Michalski AI, Johnson TE, Cypser JR, Yashin AI (2001) Heating stress patterns in Caenorhabditis elegans longevity and survivorship. Biogerontology 2:35–44.

Minois N (2000) Longevity and aging: beneficial effects of exposure to mild stress. Biogerontology 1:15–29.

Mitchell MB, Meng X, Ao L, Brown JM, Harken AH, Banerjee A (1995) Preconditioning of isolated rat heart is mediated by protein kinase C. Circ Res 76:73–81.

Murry CE, Jennings RB, Reimer KA (1986) Preconditioning with ischemia: a delay of lethal cell injury in ischemic myocardium. Circulation 74:1124–1136.

Napoli C, Liguori A, Cacciatore F, Rengo F, Ambrosio G, Abete P (1999) Warm-up phenomenon detected by electrocardiographic ambulatory monitoring in adult and elderly patients. J Am Geriatr Soc 47:1–4.

Napoli C, Cacciatore F, Bonaduce D, Rengo F, Condorelli M, Liguori A, Abete P (2002) Efficacy of thrombolysis in adult and elderly patients suffering their first acute Q-wave myocardial infarction. J Am Geriatr Soc 50: 343–348.

Napoli C, Pinto A, Cirino G (2000) Pharmacological modulation, preclinical studies, and new clinical features of myocardial ischemic preconditioning. Pharmacol Ther 88:311–331.

Palatini P (1999) Elevated heart rate as a predictor of increased cardiovascular morbidity. J Hypertens 17 (Suppl. 3): S3–S10.

Radak Z, Chung HY, Goto S (2005) Exercise and hormesis: oxidative stress-related adaptation for successful aging. Biogerontology 6:71–75.

Reisin E, Frohlich ED, Messerli FH, Dreslinski GR, Dunn FG, Jones MM, Batson HM Jr (1983) Cardiovascular changes after weight reduction in obesity hypertension. Ann Intern Med 98:315–319.

Rivard A, Fabre JE, Silver M, Chen D, Murohara T, Kearney M, Magner M, Asahara T, Isner JM (1999) Age-dependent impairment of angiogenesis. Circulation 99:111–120.

Rosengren A, Wilhelmsen L (1997) Physical activity protects against coronary death and deaths from all causes in middle-aged men. Evidence from a 20-year follow-up of the primary prevention study in Goteborg. Ann Epidemiol 7:69–75.

Schulman D, Latchman DS, Yellon DM (2001) Effect of aging on the ability of preconditioning to protect rat hearts from ischemia-reperfusion injury. Am J Physiol Heart Circ Physiol 281: H1630–H1636.

Snyder DL, Gayheart-Walsten PA, Rhie S, Wang W, Roberts J (1998) Effect of age, gender, rat strain, and dietary restriction, on norepinephrine release from cardiac synaptosomes. J Gerontol 53:B33–B41.

Starnes JW, Rumsey WL (1988) Cardiac energetics and performance of exercise and food-restricted rats during aging. Am J Physiol 254:H599–H608.

Stevens J, Cai J, Pamuk ER, Williamson DF, Thun MJ, Wood JL (1998) The effect of age on the association between body-mass index and mortality. N Engl J Med 338:1–7.

Taffet GE, Pham TT, Hartley CJ (1997) The age-associated alterations in late diastolic function in mice are improved by caloric restriction. J Gerontol 52:B285–B290.

Tani M, Suganuma Y, Hasegawa H, Shinmura K, Hayashi Y, Guo X, Nakamura Y (1997) Changes in ischemic tolerance and effects of ischemic preconditioning in middle-aged rat hearts. Circulation 95:2559–2566.

Tate CA, Helgason T, Hyek MF, McBride RP, Chen M, Richardson MA, Taffet GE (1996) SERCA2a and mitochondrial cytochrome oxidase expression are increased in hearts of exercise trained old rats. Am J Physiol 27:H68–H72.

Tofler GH, Muller JE, Stone PH, Willich SN, Davis VG, Poole WK, Braunwald E (1988) Factors leading to shorter survival after acute myocardial infarction in patients aged 65 to 75 years compared with younger patients. Am J Cardiol 62:860–867.

Tresch DD, McGough MF (1995) Heart failure with normal systolic function: a common disorder in older people. J Am Geriatr Soc 43:1035–1042.

Tresch DD, Brady WJ, Aufderheide TP, Lawrence SW, Williams KJ (1996) Comparison of elderly and younger patients with out-of-hospital chest pain., Arch Intern Med 156:1089–1093.

Vague P, Juhan-Vague I, Aillaud MF, Badier C, Viard R, Alessi MC, Collen D (1986) Correlation between blood fibrinolytic activity, plasminogen activator inhibitor level, plasma insulin level, and relative body weight in normal and obese subjects. Metabolism 35:250–253.

Wannamethee SG, Shaper AG, Walker M (1998) Changes in physical activity, mortality, and incidence of coronary heart disease in older men. Lancet 351:1603–1608.

Wannamethee SG, Shaper AG, Alberti KG (2000) Physical activity, metabolic factor, and the incidence of coronary heart disease and type 2 diabetes. Arch Intern Med 160:2108–2116.

Washburn RA, McAuley E, Katula J, Mihalko SL, Boileau RA (1999) The Physical Activity for the Elderly (PASE): Evidence for validity. J Clin Epidemiol 52:643–651.

Weaver WD, Litwin PE, Martin JS, Kudenchuk PJ, Maynard C, Eisenberg MS, Ho MT, Cobb LA, Kennedy JW, Wirkus MS (1991) Effect of age on use of thrombolytic therapy and mortality in acute myocardial infarction. J Am Coll Cardiol 18:657–662.

Weindruch R, Walford RL (eds) (1988) The retardation of aging and disease by dietary restriction. Springfield, IL: Thomas.

Weintraub MS, Rosen Y, Otto R, Eisenberg S, Breslow JL (1989) Physical exercise conditioning in the absence of weight loss reduces fasting and post-prandial triglyceride-rich lipoprotein levels. Circulation 79:1007–1014.

Yellon DM, Downey JM (2003) Preconditioning the myocardium: from cellular physiology to clinical cardiology. Physiol Rev 83:1113–1151.

Yu BP (1999) Approaches to anti-aging intervention: the promises and the uncertainties. Mech Age Dev 111:73–87.

Chapter 10
Clinical Applications of Low-Dose Whole Body Irradiation Hormesis

Akmal Safwat[1]

Hormesis is defined as "*low-dose stimulation and high dose suppression of certain biological parameters by the same agent*" (Liu 1989). Delivering radiation doses of >2 Gy to the whole body would lead to immune-suppression whose severity is dose dependent. A phenomenon that was observed and recorded after the use of the Atomic Bomb and was later exploited clinically in the conditioning of patients before bone marrow transplantation.

This chapter will argue for a hormetic effect of much lower doses of whole body irradiation on the immune system by presenting experimental data showing that low dose total body irradiation (LTBI) can enhance the immune system's capabilities to recognize and attack cancer cells. A hypothesis suggesting that this "hormetic" immune enhancement is responsible for the clinical therapeutic results that are observed after LTBI will be presented. This hypothesis is supported by experimental studies and by the interesting observation that the clinical therapeutic effect of LTBI has a hormetic pattern, i.e., it is lost at high radiation doses. This is illustrated in Fig. 1.

It is important here to emphasize that possible immune enhancement of low doses of irradiation is not a "beneficial effect" of low dose irradiation. The description "beneficial effects" is hardly a scientific term and it is important here to remember that LTBI may increase the risk of secondary leukaemia after long observation periods (Travis et al. 1996; Travis et al. 1994; Travis et al. 1993; Travis et al. 1991). The data and arguments in this chapter should not therefore be used for, or interpreted as, a support for calls to loosen up radiation protection rules and guidelines.

Historical Background and Introduction

The first therapeutic total body irradiation (TBI) in the 1920s and 1930s, was, by our current practice and definition of dose delivery, a low-dose irradiation. The radiation dose delivered were fractions of the 'erythema dose' that was repeated

[1]Oncology Department, Aarhus University Hospital, Denmark and Radiotherapy Department, National Cancer Institute, Cairo University, Egypt.

E. Le Bourg and S.I.S. Rattan (eds.), *Mild Stress and Healthy Aging.*

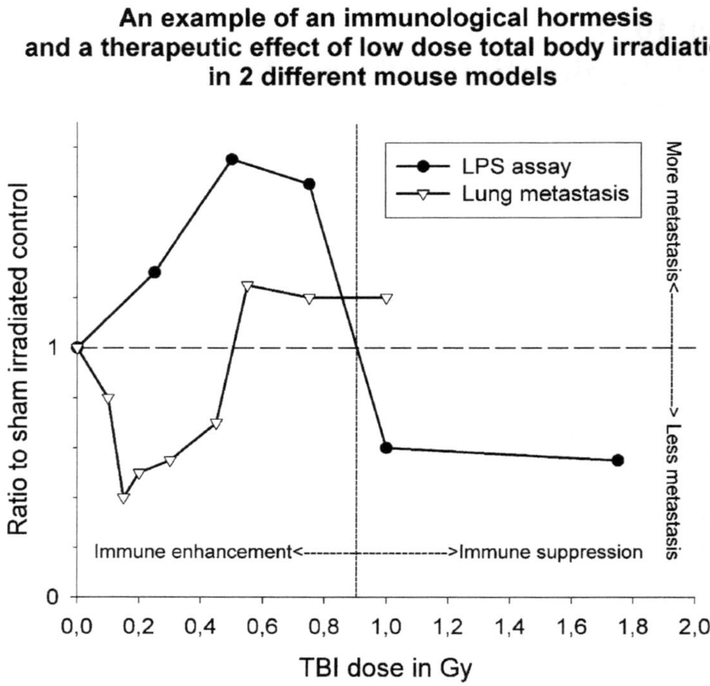

Fig. 1 Data from two separate studies. The line with closed circles shows a typical hormetic immunological phenomenon with enhanced proliferation of splenocytes from whole body irradiated mice (relative to un-irradiated controls) using the lipo-polysaccharide (LPS) assay. Maximum enhancement occurred between 0.4–0.6 Gy followed by immune-suppression (Liu et al. 1994b). The line with open triangles shows reduction of lung metastasis by low dose irradiation (relative to un-irradiated controls) given to mice injected with Lewis Lung Carcinoma cells (Hosoi and Sakamoto 1993). Similar to the hormetic pattern of immune enhancement, the therapeutic effects of low dose irradiation is lost at higher doses

twice weekly until there was an appreciable fall in the peripheral white cells and/or platelets count (Heublein 1932). With this type of treatment it is estimated that the maximum dose that was delivered could not have exceeded 3 Gy and that the dose per fraction was in the order of 0.1 Gy. The encouraging results that were achieved made this approach a standard treatment and the complications that were in the form of bleeding and infections were attributed to the disease as well as to the treatment (Safwat 2000b).

The interest in low-dose total body irradiation (LTBI) was diminished after the discovery of the chemotherapeutic agents in the 1950s but later revived by Johnson (Johnson 1966, 1970, 1975a, b, 1976, 1977a, b; Johnson et al. 1967; Johnson and Ruhl 1976;) and Qasim (Qasim 1975a, b; 1977a, b, 1979; Qasim and The 1979). Typically, LTBI was used in treatment of Chronic lymphatic Leukemia (CLL) and advanced stage non Hodgkin's lymphoma (NHL) and the standard schedule consisted of giving 0.1–0.25 Gy/fraction, 1–5 times a week to a total dose of 1.5–2 Gy. When used for newly diagnosed cases, LTBI gave a high overall response rate that ranged from 70% to 90% for nodular lymphomas and from 50% to 80% for Diffuse types (Hoppe 1985). LTBI was also used as a salvage therapy for patients pre-treated with various forms of chemotherapeutic agents. The typical results were an overall response rate of around 60% and a complete remission (CR) rate of 25%. The 2- and 5-year actuarial survival reported were around 45% and 25%, respectively, with the best results achieved in those with low-grade histology (Rees et al. 1980). Overall survival was not influenced by prior therapy (Lybeert et al. 1987).

Among the many difficulties that confound evaluating and critically appraise the results of LTBI are; changing the histopathological classification and nomenclature of NHL, the retrospective nature of most of the studies, the small number of patients, the non-uniformity of treatment techniques and dose-fractionation schedules, the inclusion of heterogeneous groups of pre-treated and de novo patients, and the lack of detailed criteria of response. Undoubtedly these factors would all affect the confidence by which one could draw solid conclusions (Safwat 2000b).

Recent studies, however, can still confirm the effectiveness of LTBI. In a study by Richaud et al. in 1998, 26 patients with newly diagnosed localized (stage I–II) low-grade NHL were treated with two courses of TBI of 0.75 Gy each followed 4 weeks later by involved-field (IF) irradiation (40 Gy in 20 fractions). Twenty-four patients achieved complete remission (CR) after LTBI and all patients except one were in CR after the localized IF irradiation. Nineteen patients remain alive and disease-free with a median follow up of 52.6 months. These results initiated a new EORTC clinical trial comparing involved field radiotherapy with LTBI + IF in stage I–II low-grade NHL (Richaud et al. 1998). Our own recent study in a group of 35 patients with relapsed and/or chemo-resistant non-Hodgkin's lymphoma (NHL) showed that, LTBI + involved-field radiotherapy to bulky sites achieved a complete remission rate of 29%, 2-year progression-free survival of 32% and a median progression-free survival of 12 months. The 2-year survival was 42% and the median survival was 17 months (Safwat et al. 2003b).

The problem here is that standard radiobiological knowledge of radiation induced direct cell kill whether by apoptosis or as a result of DNA double strand breaks can't explain these results (Safwat 2000a) because (a) response rate is higher than what could be explained by our knowledge of lymphoma radiosensitivity; (b) the data do not show dose–response relationship (no value of LTBI doses >1.5 Gy) which defies the conventional wisdom that more (dose) is better; and finally (c) no effect of overall treatment time, i.e., a short course of 10 daily fractions over 12 days is not less effective than a long protracted course of a few weeks (Dijk-Milatz 1979).

One of the theories put forward to explain the efficacy of low-dose TBI is that it could be partly attributed to a radiation-induced immune enhancement rather than to direct killing of tumor cells by radiation (Safwat 2000a). If this theory is proved to be true, the use of low dose TBI would perhaps be the first example of the use of hormesis in therapy.

Tumour and Immunity

Traditional immunology textbooks (Ivan Roitt 1997) explain that tumors can induce immune responses that are both innate and acquired. Innate immune mechanisms are significant in this regard with two major players namely Macrophages and Natural Killer (NK) cells. Macrophages, which often infiltrate a tumor mass, can destroy tumor cells in tissue culture when activated by a variety of factors that include interferon-γ (INF-γ). On the other hand, resting and Interleukin-2 (IL-2)-activated NK cells are cytolytic for certain tumor targets. The antitumor effects of acquired immunity are thought to be mediated through the cytotoxic T cells. Activation of cytotoxic cells starts with the activation and proliferation of T-helper cells, a process that is critically dependent on the synthesis of IL-2 receptors and the production of IL-2 and that will encourage the development of TH1 cells, on the expense of the TH2 cells. In a TH1 mediated pathway the activated T-helper cells will stimulate precursors of cytotoxic T cells to proliferate and differentiate into cytotoxic T cells through secretion of IL-2, IL-6, Inf-γ and tumor necrosis factor β (TNF-β) cytokines(34). A diagramatic summary of these mechanisms and pathways is seen in Fig. 2.

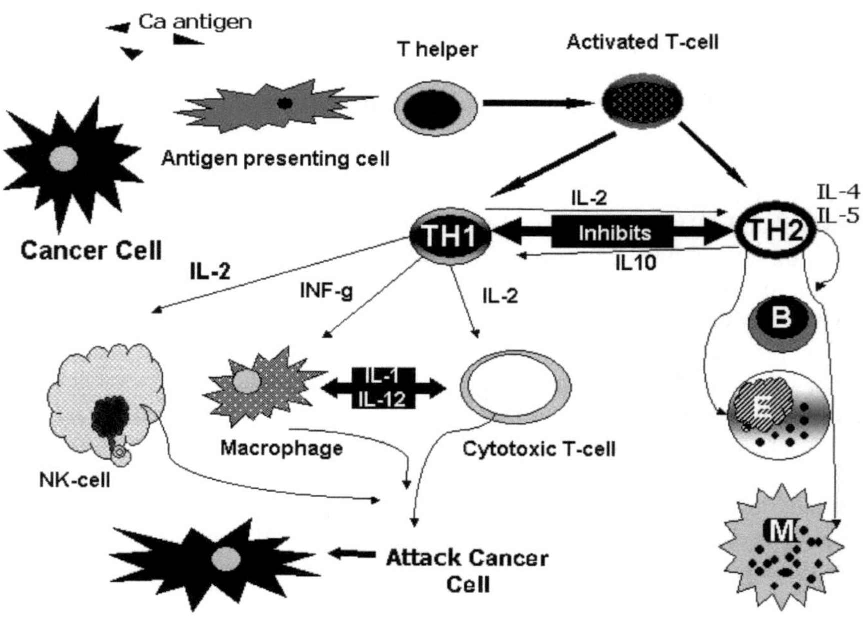

Fig. 2 A simplified diagrammatic representation of the cascade of immunological events that leads to initiation of anti-tumour TH1 immunity. Main players are natural killer (NK) cells, Macrophages and the cytotoxic T cells while the key cytokines are Interleukin (IL) IL-1, IL-12, IL-2 and interferon gamma (INF-g). Cells stimulated in the TH2 pathway are B-cells Lymhocytes (B), Eisiophils (E) and Monocytes (M)

The activation of cytotoxic cells could be suppressed by the transforming growth factor β (TGF- β) secreted by the T-suppressor cells (and some tumor cells). This suppression occurs through blocking IL-2-induced proliferation of T-helper cells. This same suppression could also be triggered by the vast array of antigens produced by tumor cells (Ivan Roitt 1997).

Immune enhancement could thus be induced by two mechanisms: an augmentation of the immune response through direct and/or indirect stimulation of the TH1 pathway (cells and cytokines) and/or a differential elimination of the T-suppressor subset of lymphocytes.

LTBI-Induced Immune-Enhancement in Humans

It is unfortunate that none of the old clinical studies actually addressed the question of how LTBI works. One can however see circumstantial evidence and theoretical support for the idea in the fact that LTBI is most effective in indolent lymphomas that is known to respond to immune modulation and immunetherapy. Another, indirect evidence could be drawn from the lack additive effect of combining LTBI with the immune-suppressive chemotherapy in lymphomas and CLL (Leimert et al. 1979; Roncadin et al. 1991; Roncadin et al. 1994; Young et al. 1977).

In an old but insightful clinical study, nine non-Hodgkin's lymphoma patients for whom previous chemotherapy had failed were treated with fractionated low-dose TBI (1.2–1.8 Gy). Peripheral blood samples were taken prior to, during and after scheduled therapy, and tested for the number of peripheral blood B cells using the EAC (sheep erythrocytes coated with antibody and complement) and E (sheep erythrocytes) rosetting cell assays. The cells were also tested for the proliferative responses to Con A, PHA and pokeweed mitogens. The study showed that LTBI appeared to enhance rather than suppress the *in vitro* immune response in several patients. The altered numbers and percentages of B and T cells in peripheral blood were correlated neither with the clinical findings nor with the treatment outcome. However, mitogen responses were 127–319% of the initial values for all five patients with complete response. By contrast, mitogen responses were not improved in the patients with unchanged or progressive disease. Thus clinical improvement correlated with the appearance or increase of mitogen-induced proliferative responses but not with changes in the percentages of B-cell populations (Yonkosky et al. 1978). Though this study did not prove that these immune-enhancing effects were responsible for the clinical outcome (since correlation does not necessary mean causation), it was very important in demonstrating that low-dose TBI could cause a certain degree of immune enhancement in humans.

Another study has analyzed the peripheral blood lymphocytes in patients with advanced cancer or NHL who received LTBI. The results indicated that the proportion of the suppressor-inducer T lymphocytes and suppressor T lymphocytes appeared to decrease slightly while the proportion of cytotoxic T lymphocytes, helper-inducer T lymphocytes and helper T lymphocytes, increased during LTBI (Takai et al. 1989).

In a group of 14 patients with relapsed and/or chemo-resistant NHL, who received LTBI we have looked at the immuno-staining and flow cytometry of peripheral and found that LTBI lead to a significant increase in the percentage of CD4+ cells with a consequent significant increase in the CD4+/CD8+ ratio. High lymphocytic percent and a high percentage of CD4+ cells before LTBI were significantly correlated with longer response duration and overall survival. These data points to immune enhancement as a possible mechanism and may suggest that the pre-treatment percentage of lymphocytes and CD4+ cells may be used as predictors for response to LTBI (Safwat et al. 2003b).

Studies of the immune system of A-bomb survivors claimed some immune-enhancement effect of survivors who were subjected to low doses of irradiation effect (Bloom et al. 1987; Bloom et al. 1983) but critical reading of the studies shows that the evidence is far from conclusive.

The available data suggesting the presence of immune-enhancing effects of LTBI made some daring physicians suggest clinical trials using LTBI in treatment of patients with AIDS (del Regato 1989; Shen et al. 1997). At the same time in the EORTC trial that tests LTBI in early stage NHL, the question of how low-dose TBI works is being addressed for the first time. The relationship between LTBI and the direct and/or indirect induction of apoptosis and the relationship to t(14;18) and overexpression of BCL2 will be studied. We have suggested before that such a large multi-institutional trial could include the study of some of the immune parameters either known or thought to be stimulated by low-dose TBI (Safwat 2000b). This is because until we have solid data we will not be able to confidently attribute the clinical effects of LTBI to immune enhancement.

Experimental studies however gave a more clear and detailed description of the immune modulatory effects of LTBI.

Data from Animal Experiments

In Non-Tumour Bearing Mouse Models

Enhancing Cellular Proliferative Reactivity to Mitogen

Liu et al. have shown that low-dose TBI increased the proliferative reactivity of splenic and thymic lymphocytes to suboptimal concentrations of various mitogens in mice (Liu et al. 1994a). The same group has also shown that LTBI could stimulate these effects through facilitation of signal transduction in lymphocytes (Liu et al. 1994b).

In a series of studies, Nogami et al. have demonstrated an augmented proliferative activity to mitogenic stimulation of the splenocytes of mice exposed to LTBI (0.04 Gy per exposure per day, 5 consecutive days/week, 2 weeks). The authors also isolated T cells from the spleens of low-dose-irradiated mice. They then demonstrated that these cells possessed elevated levels of mRNA of heat shock protein 70 (*Hsp70*) and Hsp72. They also showed that these cells responded to T-cell receptor-specific anti-CD3 stimulation by producing more *Hsp70* mRNA and Hsp72 and by proliferating more extensively than T cells of sham-irradiated mice. Hence the authors stated that T cells and not B cells are responsive to low-dose irradiation (Nogami et al. 1993; Nogami et al. 1994).

Ibuki and Goto have reported that LTBI with 0.02 Gy enhanced the Con A-induced proliferation of splenocytes. However, they also observed that the response of nonirradiated spleno-lymphocytes cultured with peritoneal macrophages preirradiated with 0.02–0.04 Gy were about 120% and 145% of the control, respectively (Ibuki and Goto 1994). These results suggested to them that the enhancement in Con A-induced proliferation of splenocytes by low-dose irradiation was not caused by direct activation of splenocytes but by activation of macrophages in the spleen, and that the lymphocytes were activated indirectly. Direct and indirect activation of T cells are not mutually exclusive and that both mechanisms may coexist.

LTBI in a dose of 0.5 Gy was described to enhance the natural killer activity in mouse splenocytes (Kojima et al. 2002). It is possible that the mechanism of this increased activity is related to an increase in the level of intracellular glutathione. A significant enhancement of NK activity was found between 4 and 6 h post-irradiation which coincided with the changes in the glutathione levels in mouse splenocytes (increased between 2 and 6 h after LTBI with peak values at 4 h post irradiation). In a later publication, the authors suggested that the increase of glutathione level induced by low dose gamma-ray irradiation is involved not only in the appearance of enhanced NK activity but also in an antibody-dependent cellular cytotoxicity (ADCC) reaction, that lead to delayed tumour growth in Ehrlich solid tumour-bearing mice (Kojima et al. 2004).

Enhancing Cytokine Release

Mice infected with the polycythemia-inducing strain of the Friend virus complex (FVC-P) demonstrate various abnormal cell regulatory effects such as a loss of Trp53 expression, a reduction in NK activity and a decreased proliferative response to phytohemagglutinin (PHA) and concanavalin A (Con A) of bone marrow cells. If untreated, these mice die within 40 days of FVC-P infection. LTBI (1.5 Gy) on days 5 and 12 after administration of the FVC-P lead to long-term survival (>370 days) and surviving mice had no detectable virus. Treatment with LTBI was associated with restoration of the cellular immunity. In response to PHA and Con A stimulation, lymphocytes from spleens of treated mice produce more IL-2 and up to 15 times more INF-γ than cells from untreated mice infected with FVC-P. The studies have also shown restoration of Trp53 expression in infected mice treated with LTBI (Shen et al. 1988, 1989, 1990, 1991a, b, 1996).

Studies that have examined T cells have shown that LTBI increased secretion of IL-2 and INF-γ (Shen et al. 1991a) as well as increased expression of IL-2 receptors (Il2rα, β and γ) on the T-cell surface (Liu et al. 1994b). Indirect activation T cells may also be triggered by low-dose irradiation. Galdiero et al. studied the effects of radiation on alteration of the release of cytokines by monocytes and lymphocytes. The authors noticed a greater release of IL-1 from Con A-stimulated monocytes after low radiation doses than after high doses. IL-1 enhances the response of T cells through increasing the expression of IL-2 receptors on the T lymphocytes (Galdiero et al. 1994).

Other studies showed that LTBI can increase splenic catecholamine content and lower the serum corticosterone level (Liu et al. 1994a). Through the presence of hormone receptors on immunological cells, both effects could lead to an enhanced immune response.

Both low (0.075 Gy) and high (2 Gy) doses of irradiation were found to cause sustained stimulation of IL-12 and IL-18 (Shan et al. 2007). LTBI with 0.075 Gy X-rays may suppress IL-10 both at the mRNA level and protein level and stimulate IL-12 expression simultaneously, which might contribute to a shift of the immune response in favour of Th1 differentiation (Liu et al. 2003).

Eliminatng the T-Suppressor Subset of Lymphocytes

For low-dose TBI to specifically eliminate the suppressor subset of lymphocytes, a certain differential radiosensitivity should exist between the T-helper and the T-suppressor cells. This is not easy to prove. An old study has shown that a subset of cytotoxic T lymphocytes (Lyt-1, 2^+) that can be killed *in vitro* with 0.10–0.25 Gy of radiation exists (Spellman and Anderson 1982) but its exact function was not elucidated in this early study. Another study have demonstrated the differential radiosensitivity between the various immne cells by showing that LTBI decreased the relative number of B cells while increasing the relative number of functioning T and NK cells in the spleens of irradiated mice (Fourquet et al. 1993). Unfortunately, the authors did not examine the various subsets of T cells. So, while evidence that a differential sensitivity exists between the T-helper and the T-suppressor cells is not proved, the idea itself is not totally refutable (Safwat 2000a).

In Tumour Bearing Mouse Models

A Japanese group showed that the growth of implanted KDH-8 hepatoma in the hind limbs of rats was suppressed for 7 days after 0.2 Gy of LTBI and that spontaneous metastasis to the lungs and lymph nodes was also significantly reduced. This was not the effect of a direct cell kill by radiation because localized tumour irradiation using the same dose (0.2 Gy) neither delayed tumor growth nor suppressed distant metastasis. Moreover, the groups conducted another experiment in which the animals were irradiated to the whole body while their lungs were shielded with 5 cm lead blocks. The suppression of lung metastasis by LTBI was the same for both shielded and unshielded groups. This excluded that the suppression of metastases was due to changes in cell trafficking caused by radiation-induced inflammatory reaction in the lungs, the authors concluded that "LTBI brought about anti-tumour effects through host immune response, unlike those produced by high dose irradiation". They also showed that, in contrast to localized irradiation, LTBI of 0.2 Gy led to a significant increase in the tumor tissue-infiltrating lymphocytes ($P < 0.01$) (64) and that in splenocytes, mRNA expression of the genes that encode INF-γ and TNF-α increased, while that of TGF-β decreased. They found no expression of mRNA of the genes of cytokines selectively driving differentiation of the undesirale TH2 differentiation (IL-4, IL-6 and IL-10). The authors also proved that the mRNA for the genes that encode these cytokines was likely to be derived from normal cells in the host animal (Hashimoto 1997; Hashimoto et al. 1999).

In another tumour model BALB/c mice were irradiated with single doses of 0.1 or 0.2 Gy TBI and injected intravenously 2 h later with syngeneic L1 sarcoma cells. The numbers of pulmonary metastasis were significantly reduced in the irradiated mice compared to sham-irradiated controls. At the same time, a significant stimulation of NK cell-mediated cytotoxic activity was detected in splenocyte suspensions obtained from irradiated mice compared to sham-irradited controls. When NK response was suppressed by intraperitoneal injection of anti-asialo GM1 antibody, the anti-tumour effect of LTBI was totally abrogated (Cheda et al. 2004).

The Hormetic Dose and Time Responses

Immune-enhancing effects were detected with doses as low as 0.02 Gy with some evidence of a dose–response relationship showing greater response with increasing dose (Ibuki and Goto 1994) over a relatively narrow window. This is followed by a reversal of the immune-enhancement effect with higher doses leading to cell depletion and immune suppression. An example is seen in the reactivity of mouse thymocytes to IL-1 which was described to increase between 0.025 and 0.1 Gy but decrease when higher doses (0.25 Gy) were given (Liu et al. 1987; Liu 2003). Similarly, Con A-induced proliferation of spleno-lymphocytes was enhanced by 0.02 Gy irradiation but inhibited by 0.2 Gy. This dose range at which immune enhancement occurs is probably dependent on the animal strain and the end point being tested. The dependence on other factors such as the dose rate or fractioantion is poorly investigated.

Unfotunately most of the studies in the literature were not designed to study the time–response relationship of immune enhancement induced by LTBI. Available data suggests that some of the immune enhancement and antitumor effects induced by LTBI are short-lived and last for few hours (e.g., splenic NK and peritoneal macrophage stimulation lasts less than 12 h) (Kojima et al. 2002; Ibuki and Goto 1994), while others, such as the increased secretion of INF-γ by lymphocytes, lasts up to 3 weeks after irradiation (Shen et al. 1991a). The increased expression of IL-2 receptors in activated thymocytes appeared as early as 24 h after LTBI, which coincided with the increased secretion of IL-2 by splenocytes. On the other hand, the increased secretion of INF-γ was apparent 8 days after LTBI (Shen et al. 1991a).

Combining LTBI and Immunetherapy

The combination treatment of 15 cGy LTBI (TBI) and a streptococcal preparation, OK-432, synergistically suppresses spontaneous lung metastasis from squamous cell carcinoma cells onjected into a hind leg of WHT/Ht mice and augments phytohemagglutinin (PHA) and concanavalin A (Con A) responses of splenocytes in. OK-432 slightly increased the PHA and Con A responses, and 15 cGy TBI did not increase them. However, when these two were combined, the PHA and Con A responses were significantly increased to 393% and 278% of the control levels, respectively. It was suggested that TBI and OK-432 acted synergistically in suppressing the lung metastasis and mitogenic response of splenocytes (Hosoi et al. 1997).

Based on theoretical ground, we tested the efficacy of combining LTBI and IL-2 in controlling lung metastases in a murine model for malignant melanoma compared to IL-2 alone. We found that tumor burden expressed as the percentage of lung area occupied with metastases was significantly reduced in the group receiving the combined treatment compared to control group and the group receiving IL-2 alone. This showed that combining LTBI and IL-2 treatment is synergistic and therapeutically more effective than IL-2 alone. The combined treatment caused a significant increase in the number of natural killer (NK) cells and macrophages infiltrating the metastatic sites. This was associated with a significant increase in the percentage of CD122+ (IL-2R beta) cells and NK cells in both peripheral blood and spleens (Safwat et al. 2003a). To optimise the use of this combination treatment we tested the effect of tumour burden and dose of both LTBI and IL-2 on the therapeutic potential of this treatment strategy. We showed that tumour burden at the time of treatment and IL-2 dose are two crucial factors affecting the synergism between LTBI and IL-2. The combination may not only be more effective than IL-2 alone but also less toxic (Safwat et al. 2004).

Based on these experimental data we conducted a phase II trial in patiented with metastatic malignant melanoma testing the combined treatment of IL-2 and LTBI. This LTBI and IL-2 regimen was well tolerated, however it could not be recommended because of its low clinical efficacy. No indication of increased efficacy was seen using LTBI (Safwat et al. 2005). We proposed that this could be related to the large tumour burden at the time of initiating the treatment and the dose of IL-2 that was administered. Further studies are needed using larger doses of IL-2 given as IV regime before reaching final conclusion on the validity of this approach.

Future Prospects

LTBI is a simple low cost treatment modality that despite its undoubted efficacy and minimal toxicity is under-investigated and under-utilized. This is because LTBI is a conceptually challenging form of treatment. The optimal exploitation of this modality in cancer treatment is hampered by the lack of understanding of its mechanisms of action and their possible synergism with other cancer therapeutics. I believe therefore that relating the immune-enhancing effects of LTBI to its clinical usefulness is most critical. Understanding the mechanisms by which LTBI enhances the immune system and a comprehensive view of the chain of immunological events that occur after irradiation will have an impact on the design of protocols that use LTBI in the treatment of NHL and other malignancies.

References

Bloom ET, Akiyama M, Kusunoki Y, Makinodan T (1987) Delayed effects of low-dose radiation on cellular immunity in atomic bomb survivors residing in the United States. Health Phys 52:585–591

Bloom ET, Korn EL, Takasugi M, Toji DS, Onari K, Makinodan T (1983) Immune function in aging atomic bomb survivors residing in the United States. Radiat Res 96:399–410

Cheda A, Wrembel-Wargocka J, Lisiak E, Nowosielska EM, Marciniak M, Janiak MK (2004) Single low doses of X rays inhibit the development of experimental tumor metastases and trigger the activities of NK cells in mice. Radiat Res 161:335–340

del Regato JA (1989) Trial of fractionated total-body irradiation in the treatment of patients with acquired immunodeficiency syndrome: a preliminary report. Am J Clin Oncol 12:365

Dijk-Milatz A (1979) Total-body irradiation in advanced lymphosarcoma. Br J Radiol 52:568–570

Fourquet A, Teillaud JL, Lando D, Fridman WH (1993) Effects of low dose total body irradiation (LDTBI) and recombinant human interleukin-2 in mice. Radiother Oncol 26 219–225

Galdiero M, Cipollaro dl, Folgore A, Cappello M, Giobbe A, Sasso FS (1994) Effects of irradiation doses on alterations in cytokine release by monocytes and lymphocytes. J Med 25:23–40

Hashimoto S (1997) [Effects of low-dose total body irradiation (TBI) on tumor-bearing rats]. Nippon Igaku Hoshasen Gakkai Zasshi 57:418–424

Hashimoto S, Shirato H, Hosokawa M, Nishioka T, Kuramitsu Y, Matushita K, Kobayashi M, Miyasaka K (1999) The suppression of metastases and the change in host immune response after low-dose total-body irradiation in tumor-bearing rats. Radiat Res 151:717–724

Heublein SC (1932) Preliminary report on the contineous irradiation of the entire body. Radiology 18:101–106

Hoppe RT (1985) The role of radiation therapy in the management of the non-Hodgkin's lymphomas. Cancer 55:2176–2183

Hosoi Y, Ishii K, Yamada S, Ono T, Sakamoto K (1997) Effect of combination treatment of 15 cGy total body irradiation and OK-432 on spontaneous lung metastasis and mitogenic response of splenocytes in mice. Radiat Oncol Investig 5:283–288

Hosoi Y, Sakamoto K (1993) Suppressive effect of low dose total body irradiation on lung metastasis: dose dependency and effective period. Radiother Oncol 26:177–179

Ibuki Y, Goto R (1994) Enhancement of concanavalin A-induced proliferation of spleno-lymphocytes by low-dose-irradiated macrophages. J Radiat Res (Tokyo) 35:83–91

Ivan Roitt (1997) Roitt's Essential Immunology, ninth edn. Blackwell Science, Oxford

Johnson RE (1966) Evaluation of fractionated total-body irradiation in patients with leukemia and disseminated lymphomas. Radiology 86:1085–1089

Johnson RE (1970) Total body irradiation of chronic lymphocytic leukemia: incidence and duration of remission. Cancer 25:523–530

Johnson RE (1975a) Management of generalized malignant lymphomata with "systemic" radiotherapy. Br J Cancer (Suppl. 2):450–455

Johnson RE (1975b) Total body irradiation (TBI) as primary therapy for advanced lymphosarcoma. Cancer 35:242–246

Johnson RE (1976) Total body irradiation of chronic lymphocytic leukemia. Relationship between therapeutic response and prognosis. Cancer 37:2691–2696

Johnson RE (1977a) Radiotherapy as primary treatment for chronic lymphocytic leukaemia. Clin Haematol 6:237–244

Johnson RE (1977b) Role of radiation therapy in management of adult leukemia. Cancer 39:852–855

Johnson RE, Foley HT, Swain RW, O'Connor GT (1967) Treatment of lymphosarcoma with fractionated total body irradiation. Cancer 20:482–485

Johnson RE, Ruhl U (1976) Treatment of chronic lymphocytic leukemia with emphasis on total body irradiation. Int J Radiat Oncol Biol Phys 1:387–397

Kojima S, Ishida H, Takahashi M, Yamaoka K (2002) Elevation of glutathione induced by low-dose gamma rays and its involvement in increased natural killer activity. Radiat Res 157:275–280

Kojima S, Nakayama K, Ishida H (2004) Low dose gamma-rays activate immune functions via induction of glutathione and delay tumor growth. J Radiat Res (Tokyo) 45:33–39

Leimert JT, Corder MP, Tewfik HH, Guthrie R, Maguire LC, Gingrich RD (1979) Total body irradiation and cyclophosphamide, vincristine, prednisone in the treatment of favorable prognosis non-Hodgkin's lymphomas. Int J Radiat Oncol Biol Phys 5:1479–1483

Liu SZ (1989) Radiation hormesis. A new concept in radiological science. Chin Med J (Engl) 102:750–755

Liu SZ (2003) On radiation hormesis expressed in the immune system. Crit Rev Toxicol 33:431–441

Liu SZ, Han ZB, Liu WH (1994a) Changes in lymphocyte reactivity to modulatory factors following low dose ionizing radiation. Biomed Environ Sci 7:130–135

Liu SZ, Liu WH, Sun JB (1987) Radiation hormesis: its expression in the immune system. Health Phys 52:579–583

Liu SZ, Zhang YC, Zhao Y (1994b) Signal transduction in lymphocytes after low dose irradiation. Chin Med J (Engl) 107:431–436

Liu XD, Ma SM, Liu SZ (2003) Effects of 0.075 Gy x-ray irradiation on the expression of IL-10 and IL-12 in mice. Phys Med Biol 48:2041–2049

Lybeert ML, Meerwaldt JH, Deneve W (1987) Long-term results of low dose total body irradiation for advanced non-Hodgkin lymphoma. Int J Radiat Oncol Biol Phys 13:1167–1172

Nogami M, Huang JT, James SJ, Lubinski JM, Nakamura LT, Makinodan T (1993) Mice chronically exposed to low dose ionizing radiation possess splenocytes with elevated levels of HSP70 mRNA, HSC70 and HSP72 and with an increased capacity to proliferate. Int J Radiat Biol 63:775–783

Nogami M, Huang JT, Nakamura LT, Makinodan T (1994) T cells are the cellular target of the proliferation-augmenting effect of chronic low-dose ionizing radiation in mice. Radiat Res 139:47–52

Qasim MM (1975a) Total body irradiation in lymphosarcoma. Radiol Clin (Basel) 44:205–209

Qasim MM (1975b) Total body irradiation in non-Hodgkin lymphoma. Strahlentherapie 149:364–367

Qasim MM (1977a) Blood and bone marrow response following total body irradiation in patients with lymphosarcomas. Eur J Cancer 13:483–487

Qasim MM (1977b) Total body irradiation in non-Hodgkin lymphoma and its effect on bone marrow and peripheral blood. Strahlentherapie 153:232–235

Qasim MM (1979) Total body irradiation as a primary therapy in non-Hodgkin lymphoma. Clin Radiol 30:287–286

Qasim MM, The SK (1979) Combined total body irradiation and local radiation therapy in oat cell carcinoma of the bronchus. Clin Radiol 30:161–163

Rees GJ, Bullimore JA, Lever JV, Pizey NC (1980) Total body irradiation as a secondary therapy in non-Hodgkin's lymphoma. Clin Radiol 31:437–439

Richaud PM, Soubeyran P, Eghbali H, Chacon B, Marit G, Broustet A, Hoerni B (1998) Place of low-dose total body irradiation in the treatment of localized follicular non-Hodgkin's lymphoma: results of a pilot study. Int J Radiat Oncol Biol Phys 40:387–390
Roncadin M, Arcicasa M, Bortolus R, Trovo MG, Carbone A, Tirelli U, De Paoli A, Franchin G, Grigoletto E (1991) Feasibility of total body irradiation in chronic lymphocytic leukemia and low-grade non-Hodgkin's lymphomas. Cancer Invest 9:403–407
Roncadin M, Arcicasa M, Zagonel V, Bortolus R, Valeri P, Pinto A, De Paoli A, Franchin G, Carbone A, Trovo MG (1994) Total body irradiation and prednimustine in chronic lymphocytic leukemia and low grade non-Hodgkin's lymphomas. A 9-year experience at a single institution. Cancer 74:978–984
Safwat A (2000a) The immunobiology of low-dose total-body irradiation: more questions than answers. Radiat Res 153:599–604
Safwat A (2000b) The role of low-dose total body irradiation in treatment of non-Hodgkin's lymphoma: a new look at an old method. Radiother Oncol 56:1–8
Safwat A, Aggerholm N, Roitt I, Overgaard J, Hokland M (2003a) Low-dose total body irradiation augments the therapeutic effect of interleukin-2 in a mouse model for metastatic malignant melanoma. J Exp Ther Oncol 3:161–168
Safwat A, Aggerholm N, Roitt I, Overgaard J, Hokland M (2004) Tumour burden and interleukin-2 dose affect the interaction between low-dose total body irradiation and interleukin 2. Eur J Cancer 40:1412–1417
Safwat A, Bayoumy Y, El Sharkawy N, Shaaban K, Mansour O, Kamel A (2003b) The potential palliative role and possible immune modulatory effects of low-dose total body irradiation in relapsed or chemo-resistant non-Hodgkin's lymphoma. Radiother Oncol 69:33–36
Safwat A, Schmidt H, Bastholt L, Fode K, Larsen S, Aggerholm N, von der MH (2005) A phase II trial of low-dose total body irradiation and subcutaneous interleukin-2 in metastatic melanoma. Radiother Oncol 77:143–147
Shan YX, Jin SZ, Liu XD, Liu Y, Liu SZ (2007) Ionizing radiation stimulates secretion of pro-inflammatory cytokines: dose-response relationship, mechanisms and implications. Radiat Environ Biophys 46:21–29
Shen RN, Hornback NB, Lu L, Chen LT, Brahmi Z, Broxmeyer HE (1989) Low dose total body irradiation: a potent anti-retroviral agent in vivo. Int J Radiat Oncol Biol Phys 16:165–170
Shen RN, Hornback NB, Lu L, Young P, Brahmi Z, Broxmeyer HE (1988) Curative effect of split low dosage total-body irradiation on mice infected with the polycythemia-inducing strain of the Friend virus complex. Cancer Res 48:2399–2403
Shen RN, Lu L, Broxmeyer HE (1990) New therapeutic strategies in the treatment of murine diseases induced by virus and solid tumors: biology and implications for the potential treatment of human leukemia, AIDS, and solid tumors. Crit Rev Oncol Hematol 10:253–265
Shen RN, Lu L, Feng GS, Miller J, Taylor MW, Broxmeyer HE (1991a) Cure with low-dose total-body irradiation of the hematological disorder induced in mice with the Friend virus: possible mechanism involving interferon-gamma and interleukin-2. Lymphokine Cytokine Res 10:105–109
Shen RN, Lu L, Harrington MA, Srivastava C, Kim YJ, Zhou SZ, Wu B, Ruscetti S, Broxmeyer HE (1991b) Effect of split low dose total body irradiation on SFFV mRNA, genomic DNA and protein expression in mice infected with the Friend virus complex. Leukemia 5:225–229
Shen RN, Lu L, Kaiser HE, Broxmeyer HE (1996) Curative effect of split low dosage total-body irradiation on murine AIDS induced by Friend virus: the results and the possible mechanism. In Vivo 10:191–199
Shen RN, Lu L, Kaiser HE, Broxmeyer HE (1997) Murine AIDS cured by low dosage total body irradiation. Adv Exp Med Biol 407:451–458
Spellman C, Anderson RE (1982) Low dose radiosensitivity of alloimmune cytotoxic T cells. J Exp Med 155:1858–1863
Takai Y, Ogawa Y, Yamada S, Sakamoto K (1989) [Two-color analysis of peripheral blood lymphocytes in patients with malignant tumours after low dose half (or total) body irradiation–a pilot study]. Nippon Gan Chiryo Gakkai Shi 24:1288–1295

Travis LB, Curtis RE, Boice JD, Jr, Hankey BF, Fraumeni JF, Jr (1991) Second cancers following non-Hodgkin's lymphoma. Cancer 67:2002–2009

Travis LB, Curtis RE, Glimelius B, Holowaty E, Van Leeuwen FE, Lynch CF, Adami J, Gospodarowicz M, Wacholder S, Inskip P (1993) Second cancers among long-term survivors of non-Hodgkin's lymphoma. J Natl Cancer Inst 85:1932–1937

Travis LB, Curtis RE, Stovall M, Holowaty EJ, Van Leeuwen FE, Glimelius B, Lynch CF, Hagenbeek A, Li CY, Banks PM (1994) Risk of leukemia following treatment for non-Hodgkin's lymphoma. J Natl Cancer Inst 86:1450–1457

Travis LB, Weeks J, Curtis RE, Chaffey JT, Stovall M, Banks PM, Boice JD, Jr (1996) Leukemia following low-dose total body irradiation and chemotherapy for non-Hodgkin's lymphoma. J Clin Oncol 14:565–571

Yonkosky DM, Feldman MI, Cathcart ES, Kim S (1978) Improvement of in vitro mitogen proliferative responses in non-Hodgkin's lymphoma patients exposed to fractionated total body irradiation. Cancer 42:1204–1210

Young RC, Johnson RE, Canellos GP, Chabner BA, Brereton HD, Berard CW, DeVita VT (1977) Advanced lymphocytic lymphoma: randomized comparisons of chemotherapy and radiotherapy, alone or in combination. Cancer Treat Rep 61:1153–1159

Conclusion

Mild Stress and Healthy Aging: Perspectives for Human Beings

Pasquale Abete, Edward Calabrese, Li Li Ji, Torsten Kristensen, Éric Le Bourg, Volker Loeschcke, Brian Morris, Franco Rengo, Suresh I.S. Rattan, Akmal Safwat, Pernille Sarup, Jesper Sørensen and Alexander Vaiserman

This book is devoted to the advantageous use of mild stress by animal species and humans. This is known as 'hormesis'. Various studies have shown that mild stress can be a means in animals to increase longevity, to delay aging, and to improve resistance to stress, even at older ages. These results are not confined to ill or depressed animals, as it was thought by Sacher (1977), but can be seen in animals living in optimal conditions.

Moreover, if one is concerned with the application of hormesis in human therapy, it would be of no interest if hormetic effects of mild stress were confined to invertebrates, rather than extending to mammals as well. All authors of this book realize, however, that to date more data have been collected for invertebrates and that a priority is to find new mild stresses besides, for example, exercise, that could be used in mammals. Finding such new stresses is a key to the use or otherwise of mild stress in therapy. Some years ago, one of us (Suresh Rattan) prompted a debate among experts on the use of mild stress in aging research and therapy (see *Human and Experimental Toxicology*, 20(6), 2001). In commenting on the articles of other experts, Rattan (2001) noted the practical limitations of the use of mild stress in human beings and advocated a cautious approach towards the use of hormesis in the field of aging. While this debate is not outdated, an extended corpus of new results that have now emerged in animal species make it necessary to have a fresh look on the possibility of using hormesis in human beings.

The aim of this final collective chapter of the book is to address the question of whether mild stress could be used practically as a means to modulate aging and to extend health-span in human beings. The goal is not to merely smooth things over, but to confront various points of view so as to help the readers reach their own conclusion.

E. Le Bourg and S.I.S. Rattan (eds.), *Mild Stress and Healthy Aging*.

Costs and Benefits of Hormesis

Jesper Sørensen, Pernille Sarup, Torsten Kristensen and ***Volker Loeschcke*** emphasize that, from an evolutionary point of view, any benefit is most likely obtained at some cost. In order to develop the use of hormesis as a therapeutic tool for humans we need to acquire much more knowledge of the potential benefits and costs. Benefits (hormesis) and costs induced by mild stress may partly be independent and measured in different units, so there is a potential to have benefits almost without costs, or at least with costs that do not really matter in a given environment, because both costs and benefits are environment specific (Loeschcke and Hoffmann 2002). Further, one should be aware that hormetic effects with respect to, for example lifespan, could be secondary effects arising from a reduction in fecundity or fertility, because a trade-off between longevity and reproduction is often observed. However, fecundity and fertility might not be so relevant for humans and could be considered cost-neutral. Just as for humans, domestic animals and crop plants live in environments more benign than those in which they evolved. They may benefit from mild stress since this may induce or improve various processes, such as DNA repair, immune response, stress response, refolding of unfolded proteins or cellular housekeeping. These systems could work at a sub-optimal level in benign or stress-free environments and thus a potential benefit might be available with little associated costs if organisms are exposed to mild stress. However, any therapeutic application is complex as cost/benefit relations might very well be genotype- and individual-specific, i.e., a mild stress may have a positive benefit/cost relation for one individual while, for another individual, the same mild stress may incur higher costs than benefits and thus the treatment might become disadvantageous.

Hormesis: A Kind of Epigenetic Mechanism?

Alexander Vaiserman stresses that environmental factors are a key component of epigenetic mechanisms, and that mild stress could be one such an environmental factor. Epigenetic influences, such as histone modifications and DNA methylation, can result in alterations of gene expression without a change in DNA sequence. These are known to play a key role in development. The period of early development is particularly vulnerable to alterations in epigenetic programming. At this time, *in utero* or neonatal exposures to environmental agents can result in permanently altered gene expression in a tissue-specific manner and can confer an increase in disease susceptibility. There is mounting evidence that environmentally induced perturbations in epigenetic processes are involved in the etiology or prevention of a number of diseases, e.g., autoimmune and reproductive disorders, as well as neurobehavioral and cognitive dysfunctions. These events determine different aspects of aging as well as etiology and pathogenesis of age-related diseases. Potential risks of early-life exposures to high doses of environmental toxins and radiation are well known, but epigenetic interventions (e.g., pre- and postnatal mild stresses) could also be used to induce long-term epigenetic adaptation of the organism. The cure of the age-related degenerative diseases and life prolongation might be the consequences of such an adaptation. Some authors suggest that epigenetic mechanisms play an important role in hormetic effects. For example, Arking and Giroux (2001) proposed that epigenetic effects could explain the phenomenon of the late-life mortality-rate plateau (paradoxical slowing of mortality rate at older ages) repeatedly observed in demographic studies. These authors proposed that exposure to a wide variety of environmental stressors will hormetically raise the transient basal level of expression of the antioxidant defense system genes and, probably to a lesser extent, the heat shock protein genes in the long-lived subset of the population exposed. The enhanced protection from oxidative damage provided by elevated levels of antioxidant defense system gene products would reduce the functional genetic damage associated with aging. According to these authors, epigenetic response to environmental variation, acting at the level of gene expression, would result in a reduced late-life mortality for the hormetically induced cohort.

Epigenetic adaptation mechanisms could thus be useful in modulation of the aging process. Since modern humans live under conditions of partial deficiency of ionizing radiation and other natural stressors, such epigenetic stimulation (for example those that are hormetically induced by the mild stresses during early ontogenesis) might have lasting benefits for human health. Such mild stresses may likely function as inducers of repair and detoxification mechanisms, "much as low-level antigenic challenges are responsible for enhanced immune competence" (Luckey 1999). Changes in gene expression profile have been revealed by the life-extending hormetic interventions of irradiation, both heat and cold shocks, repeated mild heat stress, dietary restriction, and hypergravity (see the chapters of this volume), as well as by geroprotector (e.g., antioxidant) action (Brack et al. 1997). It might be hypothesized that life-extending effects are most likely a consequence of unspecific (hormetic) action, rather then specific (geroprotector) action, and induced transcriptional changes may be a common mechanism for all anti-aging treatments. Some general points can be made in extending these ideas. If inducing a "transcriptional reprogramming" is a key mechanism of the longevity programming and artificial life extension, then specific interventions during a vulnerable period of susceptibility early in life could allow achievement of the optimal balance of expression and repression of various genes in the course of ontogenesis so as to extend healthy human lifespan. It seems that prenatal or early postnatal activation of some functional systems by mild stresses may have a training effect on efficiency in adulthood, and "epigenetic engineering" (Reik et al. 2003) could play an important role in anti-aging interventions in the future. This new way of thinking may have important implications for both understanding the mechanisms of longevity, as well as extension of human lifespan.

Hormesis: A Poorly Recognized Basic Feature of Biological Systems?

Edward Calabrese thinks that the question "will hormesis ever be used or will it only be a laboratory phenomenon?" may sound like a key question, but it is not. The reason for this conclusion is that hormesis has been used almost universally by the pharmaceutical industry for patient treatment for many years under various more cryptic names, such as biphasic, U-shaped, stimulatory-inhibitory, bi-directional, bitonic, dual effect, bimodal, compensatory, overshoot, non-linear and others. Despite the widespread use of such hormetically acting drugs, there has been a general failure to appreciate their strikingly similar dose-response features. This is the case regardless of the medical conditions treated, tissues affected, broad range of endpoints measured, and the drugs used. Further preventing a unified understanding of the dose-response is that most of these agents act via unique proximate mechanisms (e.g., different receptor pathways and receptor interactions), leading many to incorrectly conclude or assume that there is no unifying dose-response theory. Each drug or its narrow family of drugs has therefore been typically viewed as unique, a chemical universe of its/their own, with its/their own dose response features and mechanistic strategies.

The evidence to support the use of hormetic-like dose–response relationships within preclinical and clinical domains is as overwhelming as it is extensive and historically based. A detailed consideration of drugs affecting the central and peripheral nervous systems and behavior indicates that hormetic dose-responses are not only commonly employed but form the foundation for drug selection by pharmaceutical companies. This is seen for drugs used in the treatment of anxiety – so-called anxiolytic effects. In animal model studies upon which human use of such drugs is based, the vast majority of investigations indicate that the typical dose-response has quantitative features that are fully consistent with the hormetic dose-response model. The types of bioassays displaying biphasic dose responses of anxiolytic behaviors include the full range of standard drug screening studies such as the elevated-plus maze test, the open-field test, the light-dark test, the stair climbing test, forced swimming test, numerous conflict tests, the hole board test and others. Thus, in the case of anxiety-reducing drugs, hormetic dose-responses in screening studies are a necessary prelude before proceeding to clinical trials.

What is true for anxiolytic drugs is also the case for Alzheimer's disease (AD) drugs. In fact, all drugs approved for use by the US Food and Drug Administration for memory improvement in AD patients display the hormetic-like biphasic dose–response relationship. The historical foundations of memory-enhancing drugs that led to the development of the current set of AD drugs is founded on research that originated in the 1960s at the University of California, Berkeley, starting with the drug physostigmine, which also displayed clear evidence of a hormetic dose response.

This is also the case with respect to anti-seizure medications for epilepsy and related conditions. In this case, the hormetic dose-response has been documented copiously. Low doses of effective anti-seizure drugs increase the thresholds of seizure-inducing drugs in preclinical animal model screening tests, thereby reducing the risk of seizures. At higher doses these drugs increase the risk of seizures leading to the inverted U-shaped dose-response when plotted across a broad dose range. An analysis of the dose response features of these anti-seizure drugs clearly conforms to the quantitative features of the hormetic dose-response.

The hormetic effect is also apparent in the use of anti-pain medications, including that seen in drugs such as the opioids, but also for other chemical classes as well. In addition, hormetic dose-responses influence the selection of doses used in the prevention of nausea and vomiting in cancer chemotherapies.

Several dozen drugs reduce stroke-induced damage via hormetic processes. All display the typical U-shaped dose-response. These findings have been reported in animal models. While the vast majority of these drugs have not yet been approved for clinical use, this is not an argument against the implementation of the hormetic concept, but rather is a reflection of the inherent difficulties in transitioning from the laboratory to the clinic, especially in the case of stroke medications.

The concept of preconditioning in the biomedical sciences is another example of hormesis (Calabrese et al. 2007; see also the chapter by Abete and Rengo). This concept is being implemented in various aspects of clinical practice, especially tissue/organ transplants. The concept of hormesis is also seen epidemiologically in that individuals with angina pain who have a subsequent heart attack display significantly less heart damage than individuals not experiencing the prior hypoxic stress.

Hormesis is currently being applied widely in the biomedical sciences. Despite the enormous usage of the concept and its successes, many in the biomedical community have not considered hormetic effects, especially when the response is outside of the therapeutic zone. For example, in the case of anti-tumor drugs, the goal is to kill the tumor cell. However, it is now known that a large proportion of antitumor drugs act hormetically by enhancing the proliferation of tumor drugs at low concentrations (Calabrese 2005). This may place the patient at risk when the drug titer decreases into the hormetic zone. That low doses of anti-tumor agents routinely stimulate tumor cells at low doses is not widely appreciated and is probably never considered in patient management, either in theory or in practice. This management failure in practice when using anti-tumor drugs also occurs in the use of antibiotics and anti-viral agents. This indicates that the biomedical/clinical scientists can "see" hormetic effects when they "solve" their problem, but do not anticipate it when the response is outside of their normal purview. This suggests the absence of a coherence theory of the dose response to guide and influence the biological and biomedical sciences. Thus, despite considerable progress in the use of hormesis in drug discovery, development and in the clinic, much more progress is needed.

The failure to recognize that the hormetic dose-response is a basic feature of biological system responsiveness, rather than a perpetual series of serendipitous discoveries by surprised investigators, has important implications. These include issues relating to animal model selection (e.g., background disease incidence, endpoint variability), number and spacing of doses, clinical implications of a hormetic-limited ceiling effect, estimated width of the therapeutic zone and other factors. Thus, the real question is not when will hormesis be used in clinical practice, but when will it be seen as a basic principle in the biomedical sciences that can *a priori* guide and enlighten decision making in the clinical and public health domains. However, unbridled hyper-specialization and its impact on the creation of numerous terms for the same basic concept and a continuing lack of scientific intellectual leadership remain powerful obstacles that will continue to impede a speedier impact of hormesis on the medical community and public health.

Modifying Safety Regulations?

For ***Edward Calabrese***, the field of risk assessment has long been dominated by the use of the threshold dose-response model for application to non-carcinogen risk assessment and the linearity-at-low-dose model for application to carcinogen risk assessment. The application of these models, especially the linearity-at-low-dose model, is widely believed to be very conservative in estimation of risk and is, moreover, not verifiable (Calabrese 2004). Regulatory agencies, such as the US Environmental Protection Agency (EPA), have been only interested in the possibility of toxic effects and in their prevention. In contrast, environmental agencies have not been interested in health promotion, even to the point of denial that such effects could be induced by chemical/physical stressor agents. That environmental regulatory agencies are only interested in preventing disease may appear to represent a positive perspective, but it can have important negative public health consequences. For example, if a J-shaped dose response were present the optimal population exposure point would be at the nadir of the J. Yet, agencies like the US EPA and their counterparts in essentially all other western countries, continue to push for doses that are progressively lower, even when the risk curve turns upward and where the costs for further clean up becomes progressively accelerated. These actions reflect a protectionist perspective that is philosophically founded, yet not data driven. It is a perspective that continues to place blind faith in a linear-at-low-dose model that can never be tested (e.g., risks of less than 1 in 1,000 can not be tested in the laboratory nor assessed epidemiologically). Nor can they be validated, but must be 'believed' and thereby accepted. In this sense there is a complete disconnection between the actions of environmental regulatory agencies and those of the pharmaceutical industry, which must demonstrate practical results. In the short term there is little likelihood that governmental regulatory agencies will have the political support and intellectual leadership to consider objectively the entire dose-response continuum and how the hormesis concept could be formally incorporated into the risk assessment process in western countries. However, this situation could change if a country such as China were to adopt hormesis as the default model in its risk assessment practices. This could lead to much lower costs for goods and services, giving it a significant advantage in the marketplace while improving public health. If this were to occur it could lead to a re-examination of hormesis in western countries in order to enhance economic competitiveness. Short of some type of external condition such as the hypothetical China scenario, there is little likelihood for a hormesis revolution in the environmental domain, even though the scientific basis for it has become progressively stronger and intellectually convincing. A significant drop in economic competitiveness in the USA and other western countries that is related to excessive environmental regulations is likely to provide the "learning moment" that will lead elected officials in the west to conclude that it may be time for hormesis to guide environmental agencies.

The point of view stated by Edward Calabrese is controversial, because other authors do not share it. ***Brian Morris***, while appreciating certain aspects of the biological phenomenon of hormesis, emphasizes that the assumption that hormesis is generally adaptive could be an oversimplification of the complex biological processes involved. "Even if certain low-dose effects were sometimes considered beneficial, this should not influence regulatory decisions to allow increased environmental exposures to toxic and carcinogenic agents, given factors such as inter-individual differences in susceptibility and multiplicity in exposures" (Thayer et al. 2005). Thus, as a general principle, the potential adverse consequences of instituting policies based on low-dose beneficial effects means we must end with a note of caution pending the outcome of much more research in this fascinating area. ***Éric Le Bourg*** emphasizes that the adoption of the hormetic model by environmental regulatory agencies could allow them to raise the current safe level of chemicals or various forms of radiation in the environment, since low doses would be considered as non-toxic and even *beneficial* to public health (Thayer et al. 2006). The benefit of such a view for, for example, chemical or tobacco companies is of potential concern, since there is a risk that these companies could try to distort the scientific debate on hormesis. There is no reason to adopt a balanced view when public health is concerned and all other questions, such as economic competitiveness, expected profits, values of stocks in Wall Street are then of a minor importance. For the time being, it seems wise not to adopt the hormetic model in safety regulations because opening a Pandora's box is easy, but closing it is another story.

Using Hormesis in Therapy: General Issues

Suresh Rattan emphasizes that since hormetic effects of mild stress are quite moderate, it may be difficult to envisage their application as an intervention in human aging and disease prevention. However, it should be pointed out that although the initial hormetic effects may be relatively small when studied at the level of an individual biochemical step, often the final biological outcome, such as overall stress-tolerance, functional improvement and survival, is much larger, synergistic and pleiotropic. This suggests that hormesis would be involved in the biological amplification of adaptive responses leading to the improvement in overall cellular function and performance. Exercise is a good example of where it is not only the specific muscle targets which gain benefit from mild stress, but improvements in the immune system, cardiovascular system, sex hormones, libido and mood, as are well documented (see the chapter by Ji).

At present there is little knowledge concerning the interactive molecular pathways which, through a process of biological amplification, result in the maintenance and/or improvement of physiological function. Furthermore, in the case of human beings, the role of mental state and psychological challenge in modulating various physiological functions, such as the immune response, stress hormone synthesis, gene expression, cardiac output and muscle strength are only beginning to be addressed.

The main promise and potential of hormesis as a modulator of aging lies in its mode of action. Since hormetic effects involve a series of molecular and physiological processes, the final target of hormesis is the overall homeodynamic machinery of living systems. Although hormesis-inducing stress may be targeted at a single pathway, the cascade of biological effects and their amplification results in the modulation and strengthening of total homeodynamic ability.

Although resolution of these issues will require much more research on hormesis than that being done at present, analyses of the published data and new experiments performed with a variety of biological systems using a range of physical, chemical and biological stressors have clearly put hormesis on a solid footing. In the context of modulating aging, repeated mild stress-induced hormesis increases the boundaries of the homeodynamic space, thus giving cells and organisms wider margins for metabolic fluctuation and adaptation. Increased efficiency of maintenance and repair pathways, and decreased molecular heterogeneity, are two of the major hallmarks of improved homeodynamics. Hormesis can slow down the rate and extent of shrinkage of the homeodynamic space, and can prevent the onset and/or decrease the intensity of age-related impairments and of diseases. The scientific foundations of hormesis are now strong enough to build upon.

Brian Morris stresses that although the significance of hormesis is beginning to be appreciated (see the chapter by Calabrese), the use of hormetic principles in health care are controversial (Thayer et al. 2005). Scientific support for the hormetic nonmonotonic dose-response curve is extensive. As a recent example, the large US National Cancer Institute antitumor drug screening database demonstrates that effects from low-level exposures are inconsistent with the threshold model and are instead supportive of the hormetic model (Cook and Calabrese 2006). Indeed, the threshold Dose-Response Model has now been officially "buried" (Calabrese 2007) and it has been suggested that toxicology should address regulatory issues surrounding the risk-benefit of low-dose effects (see above the Calabrese's comments, but also those of Le Bourg).

Hormetic effects are seen in proliferation of cancer cells treated with hormones or hormone antagonists (Brandes 2005). The immune response in tumor cells is also biphasic (Prehn and Berd 2006), but perhaps the most fascinating aspect of hormesis is in longevity and aging research (this volume). The actions of reactive oxygen species (ROS) vary in a dose-dependent manner. At low concentrations

ROS serve vital physiological signaling and cell maintenance functions (Linnane et al. 2007a, b). External ROS have hormetic effects (Randic and Estrada 2005; Brugmann and Firmani 2005; Le Bourg 2007). It is only at very high levels that ROS live up to their reputation of inflicting damage to cells so as to be responsible for underlying disease processes in a diverse array of common clinical conditions. As another example, the low-dose stressor of acute intermittent hypoxia can exert preconditioning-like cardioprotection (see the chapter by Abete and Rengo), and the benefits of this are mediated in part by transcriptional activation of Bcl-xL and Gata4 (Park et al. 2007a, b).

It is therefore clear that early observations concerning the effects of stressors on cells are now explicable at the level of cell and molecular biology. By noting the effects of intense noxious stimuli one can then seek out effects that are the opposite when stimuli are exerted at low levels (Agutter 2007). Future studies need to be directed not just at the cell as a whole, but at the dynamic functioning of subcellular compartments and their interactions. Clearly many diverse interactions will need to be appreciated in order to gain a complete understanding of the hormetic response of cells and thus organisms. In a practical sense, it is hoped that gaining such an understanding will assist in improvements in health at the cellular and organismal level, so enhancing lifespan and reducing mortality and morbidity. The ability of organisms, including mammals, to be able to activate their own endogenous hormetic response pathways by utilizing hormetic chemicals in the food they consume, while quite remarkable, is nevertheless understandable in an evolutionary sense.

Éric Le Bourg wondered whether there was a rational hope of using hormesis to prevent aging and age-related pathologies. He was pessimistic about the first issue because using a mild stress could be difficult in practice, as this stress must be easy to use, inexpensive and not time-consuming (Le Bourg 2001). By contrast, he wrote that hormesis could be more easily used in therapy, for instance before heart surgery (see also the Abete and Rengo's conclusions). Since this article was published, new results have been obtained in invertebrates, but also in mammals, and Le Bourg concluded his chapter in this volume by saying that hormesis is probably a general capacity possessed by animal species, which has been selected in the course of evolution. Therefore, the problem could be, "simply", to discover for each species tested the mild stresses provoking hormesis. In such conditions, there may be greater hope than believed some years ago of discovering a mild stress that could be used in human beings, if it indeed exists. More scientists are now interested in hormesis, and this fact will obviously increase the chances that they will perform the crucial experiment of discovering this hypothetical "good" stress for human beings. Obviously, concluding that hormesis is probably a general phenomenon with positive effects on aging of various species, including human beings, does not imply that scientists will in the short term be able to discover a mild stress with hormetic effects in human beings. After all, despite Louis Pasteur's invaluable discoveries on bacteria at the end of the 19th century, it took several more decades before the discovery of antibiotics.

Using Hormesis in Therapy: Practical Issues

Suresh Rattan provides a reminder of the important issues that remain to be resolved before hormesis can be applied as an effective anti-aging, health-promoting and lifespan extending strategy. Some of these issues are: (1) to establish molecular criteria for identifying the hormetic effects of different stresses; (2) to establish stress exposure regimens in terms of their intensity and frequency; (3) to identify qualitative and quantitative differences in stress-response pathways initiated by different stressors; (4) to determine the interactive and pleiotropic effects of multiple stresses; (5) to adjust the levels of mild stress for age-related changes in the sensitivity to stress; and (6) to determine the biological and evolutionary costs of repeated exposure to stress (see above the comments by Jesper Sørensen, Pernille Sarup, Torsten Kristensen and Volker Loeschcke).

Li Li Ji stresses that reactive oxygen species, generated during muscle contraction either from mitochondrial respiratory chain or by other oxidases, play a critical role in muscle adaptation to exercise-induced oxidative stress by activating redox-sensitive signal transduction of antioxidant enzymes and other proteins vital to cell survival and functionality. Signaling pathways can be activated by ROS. These hormetic effects could be an important mechanism for protection of senescent skeletal muscle that is subjected to increased intrinsic ROS generation and oxidative stress. However, there is a delicate balance between oxidative stress and muscle adaptability that hinges on redox signaling in senescence. Therefore, Li Li Ji thinks it is quite feasible to use mild exercise stress clinically to improve antioxidant defense and delay sarcopenia in the elderly human population.

Pasquale Abete and ***Franco Rengo*** think that there is some hope for use of hormesis in cardiology. Experimental studies demonstrated that preconditioning the myocardium through brief ischemic episodes before a prolonged coronary occlusion protects the heart by delaying lethal injury, including post-ischemic electrical and mechanical dysfunction. This phenomenon is called "ischemic preconditioning" and it can be considered a classical example of hormesis. There are several human clinical equivalents of ischemic preconditioning including preinfarction angina: patients with myocardial infarction and with preinfarction angina have a significantly smaller infarct size and a better in-hospital outcome than patients without prodromal symptoms. Unfortunately, the most powerful endogenous mechanism for protection against myocardial ischemia is reduced with aging. Thus, we face two problems. On the one hand, this mechanism is present in adult human beings, and therefore the cellular pathways involved in ischemic preconditioning could be directly activated by pharmacological manipulation, without the need for an ischemic preconditioning insult. In this case, chronic administration of drugs that induce ischemic preconditioning could preserve ventricular function and reduce mortality. For instance, K^+–ATP channel openers such as nicorandil and adenosine have demonstrated positive cardio-protective effects during coronary interventions and reperfusion. On the other hand, this mechanism is reduced in elderly people, and therefore a restoration of the cellular pathways involved in ischemic preconditioning would be needed. This effect can be obtained by physical activity and caloric restriction, and by the combined effect of these two lifestyle modifications in both aged animal and human beings. Thus, ischemic preconditioning can be considered a classical example of cardiac hormetic mechanism that may be potentially used in therapy. In fact, ischemic preconditioning can be exogenously activated by several drugs (such as nicorandil and adenosine) in adults and restored by lifestyle interventions such as physical activity and/or a hypocaloric diet in elderly people.

Akmal Safwat stresses that low-dose total-body irradiation (LTBI) is being used in the treatment of various hematological malignancies since the early 1920s. The usual practice is to give individual fraction sizes of 0.1–0. 2 Gy several times per week, to a total dose of 1.5–2 Gy. Surprisingly, this very low total dose can induce long-term remissions and, despite modern advances in chemotherapy and monoclonal antibodies, LTBI is still a valid option in treatment of chronic lymphocytic leukemia (CLL) and the advanced stages of indolent low-grade non-Hodgkin's lymphoma (NHL). Its use in the early stages of low-grade NHL is under investigation in a large multi-institutional trial. Standard radiobiological knowledge of lymphoma radiosensitivity through radiation-induced direct cell kill by apoptosis or as a result of DNA double-stranded breaks cannot explain these clinical results. Moreover, clinical data defy the traditional radiobiological rules by not showing a dose–response relationship, nor an effect of overall treatment time. Immune enhancement, rather than direct radiation cell killing, was then suggested as a possible mechanism by which LTBI can exert its effect. Data from animal experiments have shown that LTBI could enhance the anti-tumor TH1 immune response through: (1) augmenting the proliferative reactive response of the T cells to mitogenic stimulation; (2) enhancing the release of interferon-gamma and interleukin-2 production by stimulated lymphocytes; (3) increasing the expression of interleukin-2 receptors on the T-cell surface; (4) facilitating signal transduction in T lymphocytes; (5) increasing natural killer activity through increasing the intracellular glutathione content; (6) stimulating the release of intereukin-1 from stimulated monocytes and macrophages; (7) improving CD4/CD8 ratio in peripheral blood; and (8) eliminating a particularly radiosensitive subset of suppressor T cells. Data for humans, although scarce, suggest that at least some of these mechanisms occur in patients treated with LTBI and could be responsible for the clinical outcome of their use. The hormetic nature of these immunological effects is confirmed by its disappearance and indeed reversal at higher radiation doses.

Much is still unknown about the immunobiology of LTBI, and its clinical potential. Further studies are needed to investigate the possible synergism with biological response modifiers, and/or immunotherapy. Current clinical practice does not exploit these possible immunological mechanisms to achieve better effects. A better understanding of the mechanisms by which LTBI enhances the immune system and a comprehensive view of the chain of immunological events that occur after irradiation could have an impact on the design of protocols that use LTBI in the treatment of NHL and other malignancies. The increased incidence of secondary leukemia that occurs when LTBI is combined with alkylating agents and/or total lymphoid irradiation should be kept in mind when designing such protocols, since it may limit the use of LTBI in highly curable diseases and in young patients in whom better survival is expected.

Finally, what appeared a few years ago to be an interesting phenomenon, mainly in toxicology studies, is no longer confined to this field of research and has now entered the field of biogerontology and other clinical areas of research and therapy. Hormesis is now shown to have effects on longevity, aging, resistance to stress, and can be at work in old age, even if the mild stress was only present at a young age. These results, mostly observed in animal species, could pave the way for promising beneficial effects for elderly people and for improved therapy.

References

Agutter PS (2007) Cell mechanics and stress: from molecular details to the "universal cell reaction" and hormesis. BioEssays 29: 324–333

Arking R, Giroux C (2001) Antioxidant genes, hormesis, and demographic longevity. J Anti-Aging Med 4: 125–136

Brack C, Bechter–Thering E, Labuhn M (1997) N–Acetylcysteine slows down ageing and increases the life span of Drosophila melanogaster. Cell Mol Life Sci 53: 960–966

Brandes LJ (2005) Hormetic effects of hormones, antihormones, and antidepressants on cancer cell growth in culture: in vivo correlates. Crit Rev Toxicol 35: 587–592

Brugmann WB, Firmani MA (2005) Low concentrations of nitric oxide exert a hormetic effect on Mycobacterium tuberculosis in vitro. J Clin Microbiol 43: 4844–4846

Calabrese EJ (2004) Hormesis: from marginalization to mainstream. A case for hormesis as the default dose-response model in risk assessment. Toxicol Appl Pharmacol 197: 125–136

Calabrese EJ (2005) Cancer biology and hormesis: human tumor cell lines commonly display hormetic (biphasic) dose responses. Crit Rev Toxicol 35: 463–582

Calabrese EJ (2007) Threshold Dose-Response Model – RIP: 1911 to 2006. BioEssays 29: 686–688

Calabrese EJ, et al. (more than 50 authors) (2007) Biological stress response terminology: integrating the concepts of adaptive response and preconditioning stress within a hormetic dose-response framework. Toxicol Appl Pharmacol 222: 122–128

Cook RR, Calabrese EJ (2006) Hormesis is biology, not religion. Environ Health Perspect 114: A688

Le Bourg E (2001) Applying hormesis in aging research and therapy: a sensible hope ? Hum Exp Toxicol 20: 297–299

Le Bourg E (2007) Hormetic effects on longevity of hydrogen peroxide in Drosophila melanogaster flies living on a poorly nutritious medium. Biogerontology 8: 327–344

Linnane AW, Kios M, Vitetta L (2007a) The essential requirement for superoxide radical and nitric oxide formation for normal physiological function and healthy aging. Mitochondrion 7: 1–5

Linnane AW, Kios M, Vitetta L (2007b) Healthy aging: regulation of the metabolome by cellular redox modulation and prooxidant signaling systems: the essential roles of superoxide anion and hydrogen peroxide. Biogerontol [Epub ahead of print]

Loeschcke V, Hoffmann AA (2002) The detrimental acclimation hypothesis. Trends Ecol Evol 17: 407–408

Luckey T (1999) Nurture with ionizing radiation: a provocative hypothesis. Nutr Cancer 34: 1–11

Park AM, Nagase H, Vinod Kumar S, Suzuki YJ (2007a) Acute intermittent hypoxia activates myocardial cell survival signaling. Am J Physiol Heart Circ Physiol 292: H751–H757

Park AM, Nagase H, Kumar SV, Suzuki YJ (2007b) Effects of intermittent hypoxia on the heart. Antioxid Redox Signal 9: 723–729

Prehn RT, Berd D (2006) Whipsaw cancer treatments: the role of hormesis in endocrine and immune therapies. Semin Oncol 33: 708–710

Randic M, Estrada E (2005) Order from chaos: observing hormesis at the proteome level. J Proteome Res 4: 2133–2136

Rattan SIS (2001) Applying hormesis in aging research and therapy. Human Exp Toxicol 20: 281–285

Reik W, Santos F, Dean W (2003) Mammalian epigenomics: reprogramming the genome for development and therapy. Theriogenology 59: 21–32

Sacher GA (1977) Life table modification and life prolongation. In Finch CE and Hayflick L (eds.) Handbook of the biology of aging. Van Nostrand Reinhold, New York, pp. 582–638

Thayer KA, Melnick R, Burns K, Davis D, Huff J (2005) Fundamental flaws of hormesis for public health decisions. Environ Health Perspect 113: 1271–1276

Thayer KA, Melnick R, Huff J, Burns K, Davis D (2006) Hormesis: a new religion? Environ Health Perspect 114: A632–A633

Index

MIX
Papier aus verantwortungsvollen Quellen
Paper from responsible sources
FSC® C105338

If you have any concerns about our products,
you can contact us on
ProductSafety@springernature.com

In case Publisher is established outside the EU,
the EU authorized representative is:
Springer Nature Customer Service Center GmbH
Europaplatz 3, 69115 Heidelberg, Germany

Printed by Libri Plureos GmbH
in Hamburg, Germany